PLAYING ON THE
MOTHER-GROUND

CULTURE AND HUMAN DEVELOPMENT
A Guilford Series

Sara Harkness
Charles M. Super
Editors

PLAYING ON THE MOTHER-GROUND:
CULTURAL ROUTINES FOR CHILDREN'S DEVELOPMENT
David F. Lancy

JAPANESE CHILDREARING:
TWO GENERATIONS OF SCHOLARSHIP
David W. Shwalb and Barbara J. Shwalb, Editors

PARENTS' CULTURAL BELIEF SYSTEMS:
THEIR ORIGINS, EXPRESSIONS, AND CONSEQUENCES
Sara Harkness and Charles M. Super, Editors

CULTURE AND ATTACHMENT:
PERCEPTIONS OF THE CHILD IN CONTEXT
Robin L. Harwood, Joan G. Miller, and Nydia Lucca Irizarry

SIBLINGS IN SOUTH ASIA:
BROTHERS AND SISTERS IN CULTURAL CONTEXT
Charles W. Nuckolls, Editor

Playing on the Mother-Ground

Cultural Routines for Children's Development

David F. Lancy

THE GUILFORD PRESS
New York   London

© 1996 The Guilford Press
A Division of Guilford Publications, Inc.
72 Spring Street, New York, NY 10012

Printed in the United States of America

This book is printed on acid-free paper.

Last digit is print number: 9 8 7 6 5 4 3 2

Library of Congress Cataloging-in-Publication Data

Lancy, David F.
    Playing on the mother-ground: cultural routines for children's development / David F. Lancy.
        p.   cm. — (Culture and human development)
    Includes bibliographical references and index.
    ISBN 1-57230-142-2 (hard).—ISBN 1-57230-215-1 (pbk.)
    1. Children, Kpelle—Education.   2. Children, Kpelle—Games.
3. Children, Kpelle—Cultural assimilation.   4. Learning, Psychology
of.   5. Child development—Liberia—Gbarngasuakwelle.   6. Child
psychology—Liberia—Gbarngasuakwelle.   7. Gbarngasuakwelle
(Liberia)—Social life and customs.   I. Title.   II. Series.
DT630.5.K63L35   1996
305.23'1'0899662—dc20   96-33423
                                                            CIP

For Joyce, of course.

Preface

Although it is no longer fashionable to argue over the relative importance in child development of nature versus nurture, this was *the* issue when I was an undergraduate. My own position was firmly nudged toward the "nurture" pole in the introductory anthropology course taught by none other than Margaret Mead. Part of the reason for the decline in interest in this issue, it seems to me, is the increasing homogenization of culture worldwide—or at least the culture of children studied by developmental psychologists.

So this volume is intended to serve as a corrective or counterweight to the prevailing body of work being done today in the field of child development. It describes the processes whereby Kpelle children become adult. Not only is Kpelle society manifestly different from mainstream Western society, but its children are influenced by a distinctly different set of norms about the nature of childhood and the development process.

This work began nearly 30 years ago, and I will be forever indebted to Michael Cole for making possible my first visit to Liberia. Through John Gay's eyes I learned to look at the Kpelle with both empathy and scholarly intent. One of the many tragedies attendant on the endless civil war in Liberia has been John and Judy Gay's enforced exile.

At the University of Pittsburgh this work was nurtured by a fine set of mentors—Omar Khayyam Moore, Rolland Paulston, Larry Knolle, Jack Roberts, and, chiefly, John Singleton.

The University of Toledo funded my travel to the University of Indiana's fine Africana Library and Folklore collections.

Utah State University has been very supportive during this book's long gestation process. One enormous regret is that Carol Loveland, late head of anthropology and dear friend, did not live to see this work published.

Finally, Sara Harkness and Charles Super have been wonderful editors to work with from start to finish.

Contents

PLAYING ON THE MOTHER-GROUND

CHAPTER 1

Studying Child Development in Kpelle Society

A really major gap in our research involves the learning environment of the young child.

—COLE ET AL. (1971, p. 219)

The study reported here has it origins in work initiated by John Gay and Michael Cole primarily around Cuttington College (Bong County, Liberia) beginning in 1965. As their point of departure, they took the relatively poor performance of Kpelle children in the American-style elementary schools springing up all over the Liberian hinterland. Their working hypothesis was that Kpelle culture provided few analogues to the kinds of problems (especially math problems) that children encountered in the classroom—as evidenced by the title of their book *The New Mathematics and an Old Culture* (1967). Then they launched a second, more broadly based, study and I joined the research team in late 1967. We conducted dozens of studies of learning among members of the Kpelle tribe. Concurrent comparative research was also conducted with Americans. Children were the principal subjects in this work, as they are in the present study.

CULTURE AND COGNITIVE DEVELOPMENT

The authors identified many stable and pervasive differences in performance on learning tasks between members of the two societies (Kpelle and American). Similarities emerged with individuals whose experiential histories had common elements; specifically, Kpelle children who had achieved the fifth grade in public school or higher performed in a manner quite similar to their schooled American counterparts (Cole, Gay, Glick, Sharp, Ciborowski, Frankel, Kellemu, & Lancy, 1971). However, in summarizing the differences between the two societies, about all that could be said was that culture indeed did seem to affect measured performance on a huge variety of learning tasks. This finding is neither original nor profound.

However, the learning tasks used in these experiments were abstracted from real-life situations in the United States. Hence, variation in the performance of American subjects was interpretable in terms of reality whereas Kpelle performance variation was not. Two exceptions to this general trend were experiments based on traditional Kpelle activities— leaf naming (Cole et al., 1971, pp. 108–110) and riddle debating (Cole et al., 1971, pp. 195–197). Both experiments yielded results consistent with observations of the culture. Other experiments were not abstracted from reality because the investigators did not know what that reality was. Our conclusion serves the epigraph for this chapter.

That project was brought to a conclusion by late 1969, but it was 1973 before we returned to conduct further research in Liberia. Cole, along with his colleague Sylvia Scribner, began a study of the use of an indigenous script by the Vai people—a rare case of literacy without formal schooling. They published their findings in *The Psychology of Literacy* (1981). Jean Lave (1977) was at work on a study of skill acquisition among urban tailors. I returned to conduct an ethnography of Kpelle childhood (Lancy, 1976/1979, 1977a, 1977b, 1980a, 1980c, 1980d). I was especially concerned with the period from 6 to 13, from the time a child acquires "sense"[1] until he or she is initiated. My goal was to provide a portrait of Kpelle society that emphasized the kinds of things a typical child needed to learn in order to succeed as an adult member and, when possible, to identify the practices that were implicated during this developmental process.

KPELLE CHILDHOOD IN CONTEXT

Such practices included two broad groups of activities, which I was later to think of as "routines." These included playforms (e.g., make-believe, structured games, songs, and stories) that engaged most children and were passed down from generation to generation, and adult-guided activities (e.g., apprenticeship and bush school), which had the explicit purpose of preparing children for adult responsibilities. Most of my material on these routines was gathered during residence in the Kpelle interior village of Gbarngasuakwelle. Consistent with my desire to conduct an ethnography of Kpelle childhood,[2] I assumed the role of participant observer. My limited knowledge of the Kpelle language coupled with my informants' complete ignorance of English might have been a serious impediment had I not had the assistance, during the entire period I was in Gbarngasuakwelle, of Paul Ricks. Paul and I worked together on the earlier Kpelle study (Cole et al., 1971). Many literate Kpelle have abandoned their culture and its values upon confrontation with or acceptance into the Liberian society. This is not true of Ricks. He is, in many respects, deeply involved in his own culture. He has three wives, for example, each of whom he acquired in the traditional manner. He continues to make a rice farm every year, he belongs to several secret societies (about which he would tell me nothing, despite our close relationship), and so on. Ricks served as my assistant, my interpreter; he translated the oral material we collected, and he was my principal informant. We tended to have lengthy discussions well into the night about the material we had gathered that day, as he took as keen an interest in "getting it right" as I did. He recognized that my efforts and those of the other expatriates with whom he worked[3] would one day become a living record of his threatened culture.

I was rapidly accepted into the social life of the community. I never lacked for visitors, at all hours, and I was encouraged and expected to work, play, and get drunk with the townspeople. In fact, one of the nagging problems I faced was that my refusal to take any one of the several girls offered to me in marriage or concubinage created ill will. Gradually, I also came to rely on three principal informants: Town Chief Wollokollie, in whose house I shared a room; Yeleke, the town's leatherworker and sage; and Akewoli-la, an accomplished musician, hunter, and man about town.

I decided to approach the problem of enculturation from two directions: working backward from adult competencies, especially work skills, and forward from children's play. To that end, taxonomies of play and work were constructed with several informants using "ethnosemantic" procedures (Lancy, 1993). With taxonomies in hand, my informants led me to appropriate settings and individuals so that I could record (notes, photographs, tape recordings) in detail the components of each activity on the two taxonomies. On a few occasions it proved impossible actually to observe an activity (e.g., medicine making), so I was forced to rely on descriptions of key informants.[4] Stories, songs, and Kolon were solicited directly from individuals rather than being recorded in their natural context.

These observation sessions also yielded data on who learns and how a particular skill or playform is learned.

The completed taxonomies were returned to informants and, for each entry, we solicited information on the age and sex of the probable practitioners. We also solicited information on whether every, many, a few, or only one individual of a given age and sex practiced the particular skill or playform in question. For example, among adult males ages 25 to 45, we found that all practiced rice farming, about 50% did palm work, 15% knew how to weave cloth and one did leatherwork.

We also numbered each house in the town, then conducted a house-to-house census. We asked each head of household a number of questions about himself, each of his wives, and each of their children. The questions directed at the adults primarily concerned their work activities. The questions directed at children elicited age, birth order, school, or bush school attendance. From this initial census, all children ages 6 to 13 were located, interviewed, and photographed. Through the interviews, we developed an inventory for each child of his or her work skills and the games and musical instruments he or she knew how to play (Lancy, 1975a). The census not only furnished information on children's play and work but, by identifying each child in the target population by age, sex, house number, name, and a Polaroid photo,[5] it allowed us to take accurate random samples for tests.

Table 1.1 presents the frequency of children of each age between 6 and 13. Establishing a child's age was far from straightforward. The Kpelle have no systematic chronology and keep no permanent records of past events. Nevertheless, we were able to use parents' memory of national holidays (such as "She was born when President Tubman had his birthday in Bong County"—i.e., 1967) to place the birthdates of the children. Another common procedure was to use the system of shifting cultivation as a mnemonic device. Beginning with the location of their present farm, they would recall the location of each preceding farm (one per year) until they came to the one that coincided with the birth of a particular child. Meanwhile, we kept count of these farm sites as they were enumerated so

TABLE 1.1. Age Distribution of Children in Gbarngasuakwelle

Age (yr)	6	7	8	9	10	11	12	13
Number	32	24	42	31	31	24	28	19

[a]Mean = 9.6.

we could arrive at a reasonable estimate of the child's age. Finally, we insisted that the child be present as we conducted the census so that if the child looked much younger or older than the parents' estimate we could press them a little harder or ask them to recalculate farm sites.

The decline after age 10 shown in Table 1.1 is only partly explained by mortality. A number of children whose parents lived in the town and whose ages would put them into the target population were actually excluded because they were living with relatives in other towns in order to attend public school. There were 120 females and 111 males in the sample.

Kpelle women are extremely fertile. So many children die in early infancy, however (mortality = 50%: Erchak, 1980), that I decided to consider birth order in terms of living siblings. This seemed like a more useful measure. Hence, if a child is listed as sixth, this means that he or she has five older, living siblings. As we see from Table 1.2, the typical child in the sample had two or more older siblings. This fact becomes important when we discuss sibling caretaking.

We obtained a great deal of information by observing children learn certain skills and playforms. Early on I discovered that children in play congregated in a few of the open areas that formed a kind of square on which several houses fronted. These areas are referred to as the mother-ground and became the prime locus for much of my work. When it was not possible to *observe* children learning the particular skills or playforms we were investigating, in-depth interviews with avowed practitioners of the skills or playforms threw considerable light on how they had been acquired. The census provided a "data sheet" on each child in the target population. Hence, when I talk about the age and gender of children engaged in various activities, I am not using estimates. For every child play or work group observed at length, I determined the identity of the participants (by referring to Polaroid snapshots) and, from the data sheet, their age, residence, and so on.

Like Gladwin (1970) I learned several work skills and games, noting, in the process, the remarks and behavior of my "teachers." When learning

TABLE 1.2. Birth Order Distribution

Rank[a]	1st	2nd	3rd	4th	5th	6th	7th	8th
Number	66	61	44	31	17	5	4	3

[a]Median = 2.3.

was not open to observation (e.g., for stories) a series of experiments were used to assess the relationship between rate of learning and age and sex, transfer effects, and so forth (Lancy, 1977a).

Finally, as any ethnographer knows, just talking and interacting with people without a fixed agenda are valuable sources. I found these conversations especially illuminating with regard to the Kpelle *attitude* toward work, play, children, and social change. I formalized this approach by holding a long interview session with several informants during which I pressed for their attitudes on many subjects.

Further details of the nuts and bolts of method are provided in subsequent chapters. This chapter addresses some broader issues that influenced my approach.

First, there is the question of whether I can fairly describe what I observed in Gbarngasuakwelle as holding for Kpelle culture as a whole. In my review of the extensive literature on the Kpelle, I was gratified to find great consistency between my observations and those of other investigators who preceded or followed me into the field, who worked at other sites and on entirely different problems. The similarity between my findings and those of Gerald Erchak (1977) is especially marked given the fact that I had completed at least the initial write-up (Lancy 1975a) of this study before becoming aware of his similar study. Although anthropology has been riven by heated debate regarding the replicability of ethnographic work, notably the Redfield–Lewis treatments of Tepoztlan and Mead–Freeman treatments of Samoa, LeVine's (1984) observations on research among the Gusii are more representative. He notes that his data on Gusii witchcraft were consistent with data collected a decade earlier by a different investigator in a different village. He found his own impressions of the Gusii were also consistent across two field trips in the 1950s and 1970s. Were it not for the intervening civil war in Liberia, I would expect to find the situation I describe in this book largely unchanged—except as noted in Chapter 10—from my first visit to the Kpelle in 1968.

I have tried in this chapter to set out my methods and general approach; I also want to offer a word on where I stand epistemologically. At the time I did this study I was metamorphosing from an experimental psychologist into an "ethnographer" (a term that implies the practice of cultural anthropology). However, I did not entirely throw over the kinds of questions or even the methods I had employed earlier in research within the same society (cf. Cole et al., 1971). To this day, I continue "to forgo paradigmatic purity for pragmatic utility" (Lancy, 1993, p. x). That is, I believe in approaching cultural scenes with "an open mind, [but] not an empty head" (Fetterman, 1989, p. 11). Although this work is ethnographic, with all that implies in terms of a phenomenological, meaning-centered stance, I was opportunistic and used more direct, quantitative means when that best suited my purpose.

Another issue of importance to anthropologists is one's adherence to a nomothetic versus ideographic perspective. The former emphasizes the universal; the latter, the particular. LeVine (1984) describes these "hedge-hogs and foxes" as follows:

> At one pole of opinion are the reductionists -Marxist, neoclassical econo-mists, cultural materialists, orthodox Freudians, and sociobiologists—whose basic premises include uniformities of structure and content in human life, culture, and motivation at all times and places. They are inclined to mini-mize cultural variability and to interpret evidence of variations as surface manifestations concealing the deeper uniformities forecast by their theoreti-cal positions. At the other pole are those cultural phenomenologists who in-sist on the uniqueness of each culture as the symbolism of a people who share a history and endow each aspect of human life that appears universal with a unique pattern of meanings derived from that history. They tend to reject transcultural categories and even comparative methods as based on su-perficial similarities in behavior that fail to take account of diversity in the meanings that define culture. (p. 80)

Like LeVine, I am neither hedgehog nor fox. I believe that variation in the way societies organize children's experiences is great and that the consequences for the individual of this variation are profound. Just as I would have no hope of ever "fitting in" to Kpelle society, physically, emotionally, or intellectually, a child raised in Kpelle society has an al-most impossible time trying to "cross over" to Liberia's version of mod-ern, global society (Lancy, 1975b). At the same time, this variation does not produce an infinite variety of patterns—far from it. There are, as I hope to show, many commonalties suggesting the potential for robust theoretical speculation.

Nevertheless, the primary goal of this book is to describe and analyze cultural routines for child development in one particular society. Examples drawn from other societies are intended to be illustrative rather than a test of the generality of theory (see, e.g., Roberts, Arth, & Bush, 1959, a cross-cultural study of the relationship between game inventories and cultural complexity).

OVERVIEW OF THE BOOK

Chapter 2 lays out a theory of child development that incorporates the concept of "cultural routine." In so doing, it pays homage to the scholars who have most influenced my thinking. In Chapters 3 and 4, critical background material is offered that "sets the scene" in terms of Kpelle culture. Then, Chapters 5 through 9 discuss such broad clusters of cultural routines as games, stories, and make-believe play. These clusters reflect categories found in the literature on child development, generally, and also track the maturing Kpelle child. That is, Chapter 5 deals mostly with very young children whereas Chapter 9 is primarily devoted to middle and late childhood, with Chapters 6, 7, and 8 covering the years in between. Chapter 10 introduces the subject of social change and public schooling.

Chapter 2 presents a brief overview of attempts to study child development cross-culturally. Important theoreticians—Freud, Piaget, and Vygotsky—are highlighted, as is the role of such ethnographers as Margaret Mead, in modifying or overturning many of these theories. The perspective of human ethology is represented and drawn on in addressing fundamental questions regarding parents' aims in having and raising children. The notion of "culture as information" is introduced as one of the core concepts in building a theory of cultural routines.

Chapter 3 introduces readers to the people whose portrait is painted throughout the book—the Kpelle of Liberia. Earlier research with the Kpelle is reviewed and the principal research site, the town of Gbarngasuakwelle, is described. We find ourselves in a bustling town deep in the heart of Liberia. A brief overview of Kpelle culture identifies "forest versus town" as a major dimension underlying the cosmos. Rice farming, which brings the ordering principles of the town to tame the bush, unites these two worlds.

Chapter 4 presents an emic characterization of "work," the central focus of Kpelle life. The Kpelle define a person largely by the work he or she does (they have poorly developed notions of personality). Ethnoscientific procedures were used to develop an ethnography of work. Given the centrality of rice, Chapter 4 devotes considerable attention to the complex social machinery activated in its cultivation. But myriad work activities are indicative of an industrious and self-reliant people.

Kpelle work is also central to the goals of this study, as preparation for working takes up the largest proportion of the child's "education."

In Chapter 5 we examine the stories that Kpelle parents and children tell about each other. We examine some vignettes illustrative of the way children participate in household activities. We listen to Kpelle adults talk about their expectations for children and about what happens when children fail to meet those expectations. We watch as children imitate their elders in make-believe. A Kpelle village, in common with most preindustrial societies, is a public society. Buildings—small, windowless, poorly furnished—are used sparingly for shelter from the elements. Furthermore, most work activities are inherently social. Adult work, whether farming, crafts, court disputes, or ritual purification, is, for children, an open book. Children are expected and encouraged to observe their elders as they go about their business.

These same open spaces throughout the village and on the farm that serve as the locus of adult work also serve, on other occasions, as playgrounds. The expression *panaŋ lè-ma* (on the mother-ground) conveys the notion that when children conduct their play in open, public spaces, it is as if they are being looked after by their mothers because everyone keeps an eye on them, succors them when hurt, and admonishes them when they misbehave. With all the rich panoply of adult activities to observe, it is not surprising that a great deal of what happens on the mother-ground can be characterized as make-believe play. In Chapter 5 I discuss the process whereby children observe adult roles and try them on in make-believe.

One of the inescapable impressions from living in a Kpelle village is that whatever the case was in the distant past, when warriors were glorified, the leaders of today are "smart." They are clever and able to conduct an effective argument, and they know about their own culture and its history. They associate many of the games in the rich repertoire of Kpelle playforms with just these qualities. In Chapter 6, I describe these games and the experiments I conducted to determine what, if any, cognitive skills might be transmitted in the course of learning and playing them. One such game is *Malaŋ*, known elsewhere in Africa as *Mankala*. However, there are a number of other similar but less complicated games of strategy.

The Kpelle have a clear sense of "character"; there are those who are virtuous, slothful, evil, and so on. They also believe that these characteristics are acquired in childhood. Although the society as a whole may be responsible for transmitting job skills, character is a special concern of parents. They are aided in this endeavor by an extremely rich library of morally loaded texts—songs, riddles, stories, and so on, told to and by children—the subject of Chapter 7

One of the most direct ways to learn about an adult's responsibilities and to acquire specific adult competencies is through participation in chores specifically designated as children's work—the focus in Chapter 8. Young girls have child-minding responsibilities, young boys chase birds away from rice farms, and slightly older boys weave floor mats. One of the more interesting cases is selling. Adults do not canvass their neighbors by selling (small amounts of peppers, peanuts, other portable produce) openly. The potential for being accused of witchcraft, adultery, and general gossip is too great. Rather, young children are sent out with produce to sell and the selling process, including handling money, is highly routinized so even a 5-year-old can do a competent job.

Another, fairly obvious routine for preparing children to take on adult roles is apprenticeship. In Chapter 9, I discuss learning to become a blacksmith and learning to weave—the similarities in the two apprenticeship experiences are quite striking. Other formal, explicit means of enculturation include "bush school," an initiation process for boys and girls.

In Chapter 10, we look into a crystal ball. I studied Gbarngasuakwelle when its inhabitants were gaining more direct access to modern, Western culture. One indication of this change is that adults recognized that a third alternative (neither good, obedient child nor wastrel) "end point" to development was available. "If I show him all the different kinds of work we do and he doesn't want to work, I'll send him to school and . . . I'll let him go wherever he wants."

Kwii is a general term that refers to Westerners and Liberians who dress and talk like Westerners, live in towns, participate in the cash economy, and so on. In addition to sporadic attendance at "school," *Kwii* culture was beginning to find its way into children's play. A rudimentary form of soccer had begun and such events as the "presidential motorcade" (the late President Tolbert had only recently established a country estate near the village) crept into their make-believe.

Discussing children's initial and tentative forays along the *Kwii* road provides an opportunity to discuss Kpelle adaptation to formal education generally, drawing on data collected in more acculturated villages. It also permits me to close the circle, so to speak, and relate this ethnography to the issue of the *purpose* of enculturation raised in the second chapter.

Cultural Routines for Children's Development

Child socialization involves high levels of redundancy, where culturally important objectives can be reached through multiple routes.

—VALSINER AND HILL (1989, p. 178)

Anthropology has long been preoccupied with the question of development and change, innovation, and progress. At the turn of the last century, change and the promise of technology seemed both good and inevitable. Consequently, savants cast a jaundiced eye on those non-Western societies mired in "tradition" and superstition that failed to progress—even in the face of external inducements to do so. Equally fascinating was the study of decline, of societies that had climbed the ladder of civilization and then, inexplicably, reverted to barbarism. Modern anthropology has, of course, revealed the absurdity of this sort of Eurocentric thinking. Societies do not move along tracks labeled progress, decline, or modernization. In the study of child development, however, there is still a strong tendency to see patterns found in mainstream European–American society as the norm. Alternative patterns are seen as aberrant; thus requiring some explanation.

Freud certainly did not invent the notion that "the child is father to the man" but merely wrapped an elaborate theory around what had, undoubtedly, been widely acknowledged. In effect, children are the seeds each society plants for its cultural sustenance. Spencer (1899) was one of the earliest, if not the only, theorist to attempt to emphasize this relationship in "explaining" why a particular society—the Zuñi people of New Mexico—failed to progress. Essentially, he argued that the problem lay in their child-rearing practices, which he saw as indulgent, leading to the child's "arrested development." That is, Pueblo children's development was retarded vis-à-vis that of his own society, the de facto norm. The Zuñi failed to make much use of explicit, direct instruction. Instead, children were to observe, then imitate, their elders. Further, parents and children were discouraged from seeking innovation and change in these practices. Indeed, the traditional myths and stories of the society clearly functioned to reinforce this conservative state of mind. Our preoccupation with encouraging children to be creative, independent, and critical thinkers would have been anathema to the society studied by Spencer.

We must credit Spencer with some perspicacity; investigators down to the present have noted the same or a similar pattern of relaxed, laissez-faire child rearing in non-Western societies (e.g., Scribner & Cole, 1973). However, we must try to recast this insight in a less ethnocentric mold. The material in this book is informed by the premise that *each society generates routines for the care and enculturation of its children*. These routines produce not arrested development but development in accord with the demands placed on a typical adult in that society. I would like to try and fill the lacuna identified by Jaan Valsiner (1989a)—"The emphasis on culture as an *organizer* of an individual child's development has rarely been present in the history of developmental psychology" (p. 3)—by describing how children in non-Western societies, generally, and in one particular society, the Kpelle of Liberia, develop into competent members of those societies.

CHILD BEARING VERSUS CHILD REARING

That societies have evolved routines to rear children or prepare them for adulthood presupposes a theoretical statement about *why* people have children in the first place. Again, we have tended to assume that our reasons for having children are universal. Our society has been characterized as "child centered," we serve the manifold needs of our children. The Kpelle (see Figure 2.1), by contrast, like other agrarian societies, see children primarily as economic assets.

In a study in an agrarian community in Bangladesh (Cain, 1977; see also White, 1982), children had, by age 12, produced through their own labor, the equivalent of their parents' investment in them. From age 12 on, they continue to work for their parents, until they have produced, in effect, a 200% return, on their parents' investment. Then, after about 16, they establish a household of their own and keep the fruits of their labor. LeVine (1988) summarizes the situation:

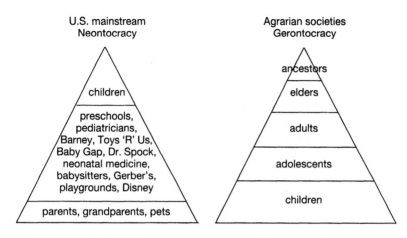

FIGURE 2.1. Child-centered versus child-supported society.

The optimal parental strategy for agrarian societies, according to this model, is quantitative; it emphasizes high fertility as its primary goal. This reflects the high value of relatively unskilled child labor in domestic food and craft production . . . of numerous progeny for long-term social support during a parent's later years, the low cost of each child to parents in terms of domestic resources, and the high mortality rate of infants and children. (pp. 6–7)

This summary describes my subjects, the Kpelle, quite well. Children are seen as making an important contribution to the household economy. Bledsoe (1980) asserts: "Perhaps the most important female function . . . is child bearing . . . , for example, the main purpose of Sandi rituals is to confer fertility on young female initiates" (p. 59).

A second, and related, answer to "Why have children?" of course, is to pass along one's own genetic inheritance but there are various ways to do this. One clear distinction made by biologists is between "*R*" versus "*k*," where *R* stands for a strategy of having many offspring while investing little energy in keeping them alive and raising them. If one has many offspring, some—carrying one's genes into the next generation—are bound to survive. The *R* strategy seems especially appropriate in the cases we are discussing here—agricultural societies plagued by tropical diseases that keep youth mortality rates high. That is, high fertility (augmented by the common practice of polygyny) coupled with a low investment in individual offspring is a rational strategy under these ecological–subsistence conditions. Further, as we shall see, the *R* strategy also influences child rearing. For example, a common phenomenon is to use older children as caretakers for younger children. A lower level of surety is the price willingly paid for freeing up mothers to participate in food production and in the production of further offspring.

On the other hand, using a *k* strategy, the parent has few offspring but invests considerable energy in their welfare, ensuring that they will survive long enough to reproduce and, again, pass along one's genes. Middle-class, Western society is an extreme example of the *k* strategy. Swedish women (Welles-Nystrom, 1988) average 26+ years before having their first child, and many will have no more. Despite the extremely low infant mortality rate, Swedes display great anxiety about the viability of their infant. It is not unthinkable for adults to continue to parent their one or two offspring well past the onset of puberty or until there is irrefutable evidence that the offspring have "succeeded" as parents. In societies that tend toward the *k* end of the *R–k* continuum, parents bear the opprobrium of society for the success or failure of child rearing. The role of parent looms large. In the United States, parents read books designed to increase their expertise (Harkness, Super, & Keefer, 1992) and make extensive use of the service of costly professionals: pediatricians, ballet instructors, day-care teachers, among others.

I should note that, in general, humans are considered a *k* species but, as indicated, there is considerable intracultural variation. The Kpelle fall somewhere in the middle of a range of societies. They are not as far along toward the *R* end of the continuum as the Bena-Bena, a New Guinea highlands group, where "children were often not regarded as truly human until they had survived for several years" (Langness, 1981, p. 14). Similarly, among the Sebei (Goldschmidt, 1976), a Southern Nilotic group in Uganda, "It would appear that progeny are desired, but children are not particularly [valued]" (p. 244). LeVine (1973) notes the widespread practice of infanticide in Africa, where children born with abnormalities and one of a pair of twins is usually killed as it is seen as unlikely that they will survive to reproduce. The attention and resources we lavish on children in our society look strange in cross-cultural perspective (Figure 2.1). As Edgerton (1992) notes: "Societies place the well-being of adults above that of children" (p. 75). Further, most societies deny the most nutritious foods to pregnant and lactating women and young children (Grant, 1991).

Nick Blurton-Jones (1993) and his colleagues have focused attention on "RSG," the reproductive success of one's grandchildren as the pivotal variable in this equation. There are three components to RSG: "production," one should have many offspring; "survivorship," one should invest in one's offspring to ensure their health and robust development; and "ORS," a measure of one's *offspring's* reproductive success. Clearly, there are trade-offs here.[1] If a mother is constantly pregnant she will have little time or energy to invest in her children; many will probably die (Scheper-Hughes, 1987) . But, it is also important to keep *some* children alive so an individual may invest a great deal in traditional medicoreligious remedies after a string of infant deaths and/or miscarriages. Once it is clear a child will survive infancy, parents and the society at large must invest in the child to ensure that he or she learns enough about the culture to make a living, attract a mate, and support a family. How large this investment is will depend on just how hard it is to achieve this normal adult reproductive role.

A striking finding motivated Blurton-Jones (1993) to consider these issues. Despite outwardly similar lifestyles, the !Kung and Hadza hunting and gathering peoples of south central Africa follow very different child-rearing philosophies:

> !Kung children are confined to camp in the constant presence of adults, yet they are allocated little that looks like "work." !Kung mothers are among the most indulgent and attentive ever described.[2] They respond fast to crying and have never been observed to hit a child. Hadza children roam about the bush from an early age, spend whole days out of view of adults, and are often sent on errands and told to gather water and firewood, or care for younger children. Hadza mothers are noisy, intimidating, and often not very responsive, and can be seen to smack children, sometimes threaten to whip them, and often ignore crying. (p. 405)

The !Kung work very hard to ensure that their few offspring survive into healthy adolescence—a *k* strategy. The Hadza, by contrast, push their children from the nest early. Toddlers are expected to become self-sufficient because mothers must nurture even younger children. Indeed, the parents' own survival may be at stake. Kpelle parents, also, view their earliest-born children as potential economic assets. These children will, from an early age, relieve their parents of many of the heavy physical burdens inherent in their pattern of subsistence, thus prolonging the parents' youthful, child-bearing years.

Thus, both society and biology dictate that we have children,[3] but it is culture that governs how we are to achieve a return on this investment. There is no universal norm that dictates a standard for child rearing.[4] What is universal, however, is the existence of routines that facilitate the enculturation—the upbringing—of children. Perhaps an obvious parallel might be marriage. All societies must formalize the relationship between a child's biological parents. Couples are not generally free to make it up as they go along. The rules, rights, and procedures surrounding marriage may vary a great deal *between* societies, but *within* a given society, everyone knows them and is expected to follow them.[5] The same is true for cultural routines governing children.

We have tended to ignore these routines because, in our society, we place so much emphasis (to the point of folklore) on the active and direct involvement of parents in shaping the child's every thought and deed. We have huge debates on the subject of mothers working outside the home and on the role of the father. The ever-vigilant parents who never miss a chance to create an instructional moment for their child are now taken as the norm, and descriptions of these parents in action have become a staple of the research literature in child development (Rogoff, 1990). Another feature of this middle-class parenting style is the tendency to engage in protracted dialogue and discussion with one's children, to *negotiate* with them as to what is to take place and how it should happen. I think such parents are much rarer than we would like to believe (see Goodnow, 1990), and even they make extensive use of routinized practices to guide their actions and save themselves the labor of constantly improvising clever things to say and do with their children. One example I have studied is the bedtime story. Parents read bedtime stories to children to ensure that they acquire a survival skill that is critical in our society—literacy.

THE BEDTIME STORY AS A CULTURAL ROUTINE

It is said that the hardest culture to study is one's own because routines and customs that in another culture might seem odd are too familiar. In effect, our own culture is almost invisible to us. However, our own "cultural model" of parenting (Harkness et al., 1992) emphasizes the individual nature of this responsibility and the manifold difficulties in successfully raising a child. Hence, in our thinking about child rearing, we have focused on the (in)competence of individual parents—indeed, the huge parent education industry is predicated on this view. But, in fact, American parents, like parents everywhere, draw on this shared repertoire of tactics. Such is certainly the case with the bedtime story. However, no one interested in child development—even in the narrow field of reading acquisition—paid any attention to parent–child storybook reading until quite recently.

First, several investigators (reviewed in Teale, 1978) found that children who were reading prior to the onset of formal reading instruction or who had an easy time learning to read in school had one thing in common—they had all been read to from an early age by their parents. Then, Shirley Brice Heath (1982, 1983) produced a stunning documentary account of the covariation of adult literacy patterns, parent–child literacy routines, and children's early academic literacy in three subcultures in the southeastern United States. She linked the presence or absence of bedtime stories to the larger culture.

Once attention was focused on the bedtime story, scholars began to study this activity in earnest (Altwerger, Diehl-Faxon, & Dockstader-Anderson, 1985; Cochran-Smith, 1986; DeLoache, 1984; DeLoache & Mendoza, 1985; Kintsch & Greene, 1978; Lancy, Draper, & Boyce, 1989; Many, 1988; Ninio & Bruner, 1978; Teale & Sulzby, 1987). What this thorough documentation has shown is that the bedtime story routine is quite complex and changes subtly as children get older and more familiar with print and story conventions.

Other social and linguistic conventions—implicated in school and in adult discourse—not directly related to reading are also developed in the bedtime story routine (Heath, 1986; Snow & Goldfield, 1982, 1983). "Picture-book reading may, in addition to its substantive contribution, be the basis for transfer to participation in the discourse structure of classroom lessons several years later" (Cazden, 1992, p. 106). As we shall see, these efforts do pay off and account, in large measure (Adams, 1990), for these children's success in school.

The cultural nature of the bedtime story was brought home in more recent studies, which document its *absence* outside the middle-class or mainstream society (Snow, Barnes, Chandler, Goodman, & Hemphill, 1991; Purcell-Gates, 1994). Further, the routines described above are not readily available to parents who are not members of this particular culture. When asked to read to their children, they display signs of unfamiliarity and incompetence (Bergin, Lancy, & Draper 1994; Heath & Thomas, 1984; Heath & Branscomb, 1986). Finally, attempts to intervene by stimulating the development of family literacy—to enhance the child's educational chances—have proven costly and difficult (Lancy, 1994c).

We can draw several inferences about the nature of cultural routines from the bedtime story example:

1. The bedtime story looks much the same in all middle-class families in any part of the world—the components are highly standardized.

2. The bedtime story is cultural because it is found only within middle-class society and not elsewhere. It does not transfer or diffuse readily outside middle-class society. It is integrated with other cultural routines that have a similar purpose (e.g., parent–child dinner table conversations).

3. The bedtime story works. Children who are exposed to this routine are likely to become literate; those who are not are less likely to become literate.

4. Given the importance of literacy, it follows that our society has created *other, redundant cultural routines*—Sesame Street, Whole Language, Hooked on Phonics—to ensure that nearly all children acquire literacy.

As useful as the cultural-routines concept is in understanding child development in our own society, it has even greater utility in traditional, non-Western societies. So many of the routines in our society share a kind of teacher/curriculum base—whether enacted in the home, in school, on the job, or via the media. In other societies, the role of teacher is assumed far more rarely and children bear greater personal responsibility for acquiring their culture. To be sure, however, the society does not just let them flounder but provides a wealth of opportunities for guided and sheltered learning.

NATURE, NURTURE, AND CULTURE: A CAPSULE HISTORY

The notion that children's development is guided by a set of culturally sanctioned routines is not entirely novel, but it does depart from the theoretical mainstream. There have been three broad phases in the history of attempts to understand how culture influences child development. Prior to World War II, the ideas of Sigmund Freud were in the ascendancy; then followed a phase when Jean Piaget's theories held sway. More recently, the vision of Lev Vygotsky has provided guidance to cross-cultural psychologists. Interestingly, each phase has had two periods. During the initial period, researchers tend to embrace the theories rather uncritically and apply concepts and paradigms developed in Western Europe in the far corners of the globe. Then, gradually, growing evidence—especially ethnographic study—mounts that undermines the cross-cultural validity of the initial theory (Jahoda, 1982).

Margaret Mead was the first anthropologist to attempt to "test" psychological theories of childhood with ethnographic data. She set off to the South Pacific with her mentor Franz Boas's blessing, determined to test the limits of Freudian theory. Freud had argued for, among other things, a universal or natural tendency for adolescents to pass through a period of stressful transition to adulthood. Samoan youth did not "fit" the theory (Mead, 1928).

Mead was among the founders of what came to be called the culture and personality school in anthropology, which, inspired by Freudian ideas, sought to link aspects of child rearing to adult personality traits (Dennis, 1940). Mead—distancing herself from classic Freudian theory—began to build a foundation for cultural integration and relativism in developmental psychology corresponding to the general trend in cultural anthropology. In other words, nature was to play a minor role as compared to culture. Societies shaped children for the roles they were to play as adults. Mead (1935), for example, documented the dramatic differences in the experience of Mundugumor and Arapesh children that were consistent with differences in the character of adults in the respective and, in many ways similar, societies. Among the Arapesh, children's play emphasizes cooperation and mutuality—adults are easygoing and considerate of each other. Among the Mundugumor, play is competitive, and younger children are victimized by bullies—a program consistent with a modal adult role characterized by spite, jealousy, aggression, and cannibalism.

However, anthropologists became increasingly dissatisfied with this limited concern for how children acquire adult personality and sought to broaden the investigation to include all the skills, knowledge, and beliefs that are part of the repertoire of a competent adult member of the society. Herskovits (1948; see also Williams, 1972/1983) coined the term "enculturation" to handle this broader agenda for human development and contrasted it with "socialization," a narrower concern for the way parents and others shape children's emerging character and interpersonal behavior or "manners."

I believe that the most important conclusion we can draw from the culture and personality literature is that when there are significant differences in adult personality patterns, they are provoked less by the behavior of parents vis-à-vis infants than by a distinctive *pattern* of experiences that persist into adulthood. Certainly a characteristic and socially sanctioned parent-child interaction style is a part of this pattern, but so, too are adult–child and child–child interaction styles, the playform inventory, rites of passage, and prescriptions regarding such things as children and work and adolescents and marriage. All contribute to building a distinct and thorough curriculum for the creation of competent adults.

The next major human development theorist to hold a dominant position was Jean Piaget, and he, in opposition to Freud, elevated nature to the ascendant role. Piaget tended to obscure this in his own writing, however. "Piaget's biologizing slipped by, perhaps because he slyly refused to take a stand on the nature–nurture controversy. Still, it became apparent that he was dealing with a phenomena whose variance was mostly accounted for by maturation . . . a fact not surprising when it is considered he began life as a zoologist" (Konner, 1977, p. 71). Like Freud in Vienna, however, Piaget drew for his theories on interviews with and observations of those around him in bourgeois Geneva, especially his own bright, inquisitive, and well-educated children. Again, the South Pacific was the site of research (Kelly, 1977; Lancy, 1983) that revealed the culture-bound nature of much Piagetian theory. We found that most Papua New Guinean children "failed to develop" according to Piagetian structures and timetables. We showed that the increasingly sophisticated and efficient information-processing strategies, posited in the theory, were of little use in societies that contained, in fact, relatively little information (Lancy 1983). Invoking Simon's (1956) notions of "bounded rationality" and "satisficing" (Lancy, 1989; see also Valsiner, 1989c), I argued that people tend not to progress inevitably to a stage of thinking reminiscent of the rational scientist (e.g., the formal operations of Inhelder & Piaget, 1958). In effect, people muddle along. When the press of information, coupled with serious consequences for error, demands it, some non-Western peoples—maritime traders/hunters, for instance (Lancy, 1983, pp. 200–203; 1989)—do indeed make use of more efficient, decontextualized strategies for processing information. However, this is a rarity. As Shweder (1984) noted, even well-educated Westerners use "primitive," inefficient cognitive strategies when they are engaged in everyday activities (e.g., grocery shopping; Murtaugh, 1984).

Piagetian theory inspired a wealth of cross-cultural research on cognitive development (Dasen, 1977). Taking into account these cross-cultural studies as well as Piagetian research with autistic (Lancy & Goldstein, 1982), deaf (Furth, 1966), and other "abnormal" populations, I argued (Lancy, 1983) that only Piaget's earliest stages—sensorimotor and preoperational—were truly universal (see also Dasen, Inhelder, Lavallée, & Retschitzki, 1978). These cognitive skills seem "hard-wired"—nature rules. That is, children seem to achieve these basic competencies regardless of what the society provides by way of child-rearing practices. As long as children are involved in a community of speaking, interacting adults, they should experience "normal" development. Second, the extent to which these basic skills are augmented by further development (e.g., Piaget's concrete and formal operations) of more versatile and efficient information-processing strategies is a function of the demand placed on adults enacting the culture. When survival depends, for example, on the ability to understand the ecology of hundreds of plant and animal species or when it depends on the acquisition of a 10,000-word reading vocabulary (e.g., a banker in Geneva), we can expect to see children "pressed" in various ways to become more efficient processors of information—nurture rules.

The last 10 years have seen Piaget largely eclipsed by Lev Vygotsky as the dominant theorist in developmental psychology (Rogoff, 1990). At least part of the appeal is that Vygotsky focused on developmental opportunities—parents providing guided assistance[6] as children try and learn new skills—that are readily visible. This is in contrast to Piaget's structures, which can only be inferred from children's performance on obscure tests. The ideas of Vygotsky and his followers, in other words, are much more compatible with the kind of data usually available to cultural anthropologists. Nevertheless, Vygotsky's theory also suffers from ethnocentrism (cf. Atran & Sperber 1991).[7]

The centerpiece of Vygotsky's (1978) theory of development is the notion that adults, including older siblings, members of one's extended family, and the community, all collaborate to assist the child in acquiring more adult-like skills and behavior. A clear contemporary statement of this notion has been provided by Tharp and Gallimore (1988):

> Long before they enter school, children are learning . . . cognitive and linguistic skills. Their teaching takes place in the everyday interactions of domestic life. Within these goal-directed activities, opportunities are available for more capable members of the household to assist and regulate child performances. . . . Children's participation is sustained by the adults assuming as many of the strategic functions as necessary to carry on. . . . The caretaker's guidance permits children to engage in levels of activity that could not be managed alone. (pp. 27–28)

Barbara Rogoff's (1990) research contains numerous examples of parents assisting their children's development. For example, she describes the "joint cleanup of a toddler's room . . ." (p. 94), where a mother painstakingly constructs an elaborate lesson in "neatness" for her child. But, by this very example—and similar examples in Tharp and Gallimore

(1988)—Rogoff concedes that Vygotsky's theory, although seemingly matched to children's experiences in mainstream Western society, falls short elsewhere. "The face-to-face didactic interactions that characterize middle-class American parents in research settings are less prevalent and may be less necessary to reach local goals in some other cultures" (Rogoff, 1990, p. 96).

This contrast is especially sharp when we consider adult–child conversation. American middle-class mothers place their infants *en face* (extremely rare elsewhere; Field, Sostek, Vietze, & Leiderman, 1981) and hold conversations with them that are structured as if the infant were actually filling in the response slot. Another characteristic of "motherese" speech is the use of a baby-talk register, with a special lexicon and higher pitch. Mothers "scaffold" their young child's speech by, for example, rephrasing their short, grammatically incorrect utterances into longer, correct phrases (Ochs & Schieffelin, 1984). More recent research shows clear links between the prevalence of these parent–child "instructional conversations" (Tharp & Gallimore, 1988) and the child's acquisition of various conversational patterns, his or her vocabulary size, ease of literacy acquisition, and general communicative competence (Lancy, 1994b).

On the other hand, research on child language socialization in other societies (Irvine, 1978; Schieffelin & Ochs, 1986) is mostly a story about the *absence* of parent–child interaction. "Kaluli mothers do not engage in sustained gazing at, or elicit and maintain direct eye contact with their infants as such behavior is . . . associated with witchcraft" (Ochs & Schieffelin, 1984, p. 279). In Samoa, "Infants . . . are not treated as conversational partners" (Ochs & Schieffelin, 1984, p. 295)."We were struck by the seeming poverty of discourse between [Kpelle] adults and children" (Erchak, 1977, p. 120). Joking relationships among adolescents and between same- and cross-sex adults are widely reported in the ethnographic literature, but the *only* reported case of a parent–child joking relationship is found in mainstream U.S. society (Alford, 1983).

Even in America, mothers outside the mainstream do not conform to the Vygotskian model. Their verbal interaction with their children is limited to the occasional directive or warning (Heath, 1990). Here is how one of Shirley Brice Heath's (1983) African American informants expressed it:

> He [her grandson] gotta learn to know 'bout dis world, can't nobody tell 'im. Now just how crazy is dat? White folks uh hear dey kids say sump'n, dey say it back to 'em, dey aks 'em 'gain 'n 'gain 'bout things. . . . He just gotta be keen, keep his eyes open. . . . Gotta watch hisself by watchin' other folks.

Ain't no use me tellin' 'im: "learn dis, learn dat" . . . He just gotta learn . . . he see one thing one place one time, he know how it go, see sump'n like it again, maybe it be de same, maybe it won't. He hafta try it out. (p. 84)

Goodnow (1990) is not even convinced of the wide applicability of "Vygotskian-based accounts of . . . development" (p. 274) in middle-class society.

My disappointment with the picture usually presented is that . . . the world is benign and relatively neutral. To be more specific, the standard picture is one of willing teachers on the one hand and eager learners on the other. Where are the parents who do not see their role as one of imparting information and encouraging understanding? Where are the children who do not wish to learn or perform in the first place, or who regard as useless what the teaching adult is presenting? Those questions were prompted especially by trying to fit Vygotskian analyses to the interactions involved in teaching children to be skilled at some household tasks and to take responsibility for them. On the surface, this type of teaching/learning situation should allow a Vygotskian analysis. It is very much an interpersonal situation. And it contains an expert who is usually eager to pass on both skills and a particular definition of the situation. Success, however, is often elusive; resistance is often open and prolonged. (p. 279)

As I reviewed literature on childhood in many cultures, I noted only one area in which nearly all parents seemed to take on the didactic role of teacher, namely, in teaching manners, polite speech formulas, and respect for the child's age and class superiors (Demuth, 1986; Robinson, 1989). Chapter 5 provides several examples.

Each of these theoretical strands can be woven into a strong rope linking culture, biology, and child development. The culture and personality school has given us many ideas of where to look in the life of the developing individual for clues to pervasive differences between cultures in adult character traits. This is the study of *socialization*. Piagetian research highlights cross-cultural differences in cognitive development, and these findings have provided a powerful explanation for the differential success in Western-style public schools of children from different societies. As adopted by those who study culture and development, the Vygotskian perspective has been particularly fruitful in directing the discovery of culture-specific practices of child rearing and documenting intercultural variation (Miller & Goodnow, 1995). The theory of cultural routines incorporates and extends these insights.

COMPONENTS OF A THEORY
OF CULTURAL ROUTINES

Unlike language, the human genome does not include a template for culture. That is, we are cultural animals but we do not automatically absorb our own culture, and, indeed, as children, we do not even have a very good idea of how to acquire adult competencies. Parents, universally, are faced with a choice, to let "nature take its course" in which case the child may well starve (e.g., Scheper-Hughes, 1989) or to invest time and energy in training children to become bearers of the culture. But parents are concerned with their own well-being, which, in turn, may be jeopardized by overinvesting in their offspring. So, just as we have routines to make it easier to wrest a living from the soil, a significant part of the repertoire of any society will be various routines for raising children. These routines are shared and they are passed on from generation to generation. Members of a society may deviate from these routines but can be expected to arouse the ire of fellow members if their deviance is extreme and public. However, in this study, I am particularly interested in describing cultural routines for child development which are carried out, largely, *in the absence of parents*, or at least with little direct investment by parents.

An elegant and formal introduction to the idea of cultural routines can be found in the work of Sara Harkness and Charles Super (1986; Super & Harkness, 1986). They argue that each child is shaped within the metaphorical space of a "developmental niche." The developmental niche includes the physical and social settings the child is exposed to, the customary child-rearing strategies, and the folk theories people hold about how children develop and thrive. One application of this concept has been in the comparative study of sleeping arrangements (Harkness & Super, 1995). From the perspective of a villager from Mexico, children in middle-class Euro-American culture are forced to sleep independently, from an "early" age. In some other societies, children sleep with their mothers until puberty. Who one sleeps with and under what circumstances may well serve a critical function in the socialization of the child. These practices are dictated by the culture—indeed, severe sanctions greet their violation (e.g., accusations of incest). The parent's schema for child rearing typically includes not only some rules to guide these practices but also a rationale or "ethnotheory" about why these practices "work." Chapter 5 presents Kpelle ideas about raising children.

A principal element of such ethnotheories is a calendar that marks transition points in the child's development. For example, the Ngoni

(Read, 1960) celebrate in ritual a boy's first nocturnal emission, the deepening of his voice, and the eruption of the second set of molars. Whiting and Edwards (1988) refer to "weaning from the back" (p. 88), an important milestone in West African cultures when the mother no longer carries the infant slung on her back. Among the Tallensi (Fortes, 1970), full knowledge and understanding of the kinship system is not expected before age 12. The ancient Greeks held a distinctly developmental view of children. Before 2, the child was expected to drink lots of milk but no wine. From 2 to 5, it was to be free to play (Golden, 1990). The Romans were even more explicit and marked stage transitions by a change in clothing (Dupont, 1992).

Rogoff et al (1975) surveyed 50 societies in the ethnographic literature and found two ages, 5 to 7 and, again, adolescence, when adults shift their expectations for children. The first benchmark is widely associated with the development of "sense." "It is when children begin to develop *haYYillo* (social sense) that adults in turn change their expectations and behavior (Riesman, 1992, p.13). Before the age of around six years an Acholi child was often regarded as *pe-ngeyopiny* ('he does not know the world')" (Ocitti, 1973, p. 47). The second benchmark is associated with the onset of puberty and is often marked by a rite of passage (van Gennep, 1909/1960) such as an initiation ceremony.

These milestones and the rituals that accompany them are among the most vital routines a society has for socializing its children. They define, for example, a child's peers or reference group. They provide an incentive program to encourage the child to behave in ways considered age appropriate. It is not only the child's behavior that is controlled by these routines, siblings and adults also have well-scripted roles to play. When we say to someone, "You're babying him," or, "You're spoiling him," we are telling an adult that he or she is failing to adjust to a change in the child's status vis-à-vis the larger society.

Most societies do assign primary responsibility to parents for the socialization of children; this is certainly true for the Kpelle.[8] But the process of bringing up children must also include provision for "cultural transmission," or enculturation. This responsibility is too broad and diffuse to be left solely to parents. John M. Roberts (1964) has written:

> It is possible to regard all culture as information and to view any single culture as an "information economy" in which information is received or created, stored, retrieved, transmitted, utilized, and even lost . . . information is stored in the minds of . . . members and . . . artifacts. . . . Human storage

systems have their limitations. . . . There is a limit to the amount of information any one individual or combination of individuals can learn and remember. . . . [Therefore, it] is safe to assert that no tribal culture is sufficiently
small in inventory to be stored in one brain. . . . [However, the] more nearly
a single individual controls the cultural inventory, the simpler the culture.
(pp. 438–440)

> . . . The greater the informational store, the more complex and efficient
the retrieval mechanisms are likely to be.[9] (p. 447)

Goodenough (1971) later coined the term "propriospect" to describe this
"culture in the head" notion and Wolcott (1991) related propriospect to
the acquisition of culture, thereby linking cultural anthropology with the
psychology of learning and cognitive growth: Children are viewed as
"storage units [that] must be added to the system . . . as older members of
the society disappear" (Roberts, 1964, p. 439).

It is easy to see how much of this information gets passed down from
one generation to the next in our own society—through schooling.[10] The
more of the total store of the society's accumulated information individuals are expected to incorporate into their propriospect, the longer, more
thorough, and more expensive this schooling will be—assuming equal IQ
and motivation. Indeed, we have great debates about the extent to which
all citizens should master the same segment of the information store and
about how to bring this about (Hirsch, 1987). But formal education is not
the only—and in preindustrial societies not even the primary[11]—means to
transmit the culture to youth. There are other, less formal but, nevertheless patterned and recognizable entities that get the job done, (e.g., games).

Games make wonderful exemplars of the cultural routines concept.
They encapsulate important "bits" of culture. Schwartzman (1978) refers
to them "as a form of social formaldehyde" (p. 328); they have set procedures that are usually well understood and there are also routines for
transmitting these rules to novice players. And, they are intrinsically motivating. You do not have to have a truant officer around to make sure children play games.

Roberts was also interested in the role of games in the socialization of
children (e.g., Roberts et al., 1959). In this respect, he followed in a long
line of anthropologists and naturalists,[12] for, as Schwartzman (1978)
points out, "children's play . . . [serving] implicitly and explicitly . . . as a
socializing activity is far and away the most common anthropological interpretation" (p. 101). Fisher (1992) reviewed 46 studies which, overall
"provide convincing evidence of the impact of play, which appears to pro-

mote . . . both cognitive–linguistic and affective–social" (p. 159) development. Roberts did not pursue this issue of "adding storage units" much further than games. In fact, he was more interested in the way games and play shaped personality and character (socialization) but he heartily endorsed the idea (personal communication, January 1972) that games might serve to transmit practical and intellectual skills (enculturation; Lancy, 1975a, 1980b).

In Chapter 6, I discuss Anderson and Moore's (1960) notion of "folk models" as "autotelic learning environments." Their folk models are similar to cultural routines and they include games, songs, and stories as folk models. The term "autotelic" means that the individual will invest time and energy in mastering this particular folk model without any further reward. In discussing play, many scholars have posited that individuals find it rewarding because it helps to stave off boredom and maintain an optimum state of arousal (Lancy, 1980b). In Chapters 5, 6, and 7 I introduce a variety of cultural routines, all of which could be considered play and, hence, intrinsically motivating.

Besides the stimulating effect of play, the motivation to master the skills of one's elders (White, 1959) appears to have wide applicability. In a multistep process, children acquire a schematic representation of their own culture and, then, of their own place in it. The gap or discrepancy between the idealized model and one's actual level of skill and diligence is *motivating* (D'Andrade, 1992). Read (1960) describes young Ngoni boys as chafing at the bit to begin caring for yearling livestock and then eager to demonstrate competence so they will be accorded herding responsibility for a small flock of mature animals.[13] Another pointed example comes from another herding society—the Chaga:

> From early days children delight in activities connected with the cleaning of the animal's quarters. Siairuka strutted about in the dung at two years of age. Girls soon begin to run after their mothers as they go to and fro dragging dung to the grove. The dung is heaped on three banana sheaths. Small girls clamor for permission to do likewise and their mothers supply them with one sheath and a small load, a measure which is increased as they grow in strength. (Raum, 1940, p. 199)

In Chapters 8 and 9 we observe children willingly enduring considerable hardship, even abuse, in order to master the prerequisites of adulthood.

On the other hand, we also observe cases of individuals who do *not* master pieces of the culture. For example, only one young man was learning to play the hourglass drum in the village I studied. Roberts's theory of culture as information is again germane. He was one of the first anthropologists to recognize that the standard ethnographic description of a society probably did not correspond to the lived culture of any single individual. Roberts (1951, 1987) carried out a landmark study just after World War II in which he inventoried the knowledge, skills, and artifacts from three distinct Navajo households. He found quite a bit of overlap but also variation. Clearly, "Navajo culture" meant something slightly different in each of those households. He made the significant point that the information contained in the society was *distributed* over many individuals.[14] So, if a child chooses not to play a particular game or the college student chooses not to take a particular course, he or she may be lost to the society as "storage units" for the information transmitted in that game/course.

What happens when there is cultural information that children do not willingly pursue, yet this information must be transmitted to them in order to keep the culture intact? In these cases, the cultural routines look like our public schools, institutions in which children may need to be coerced to attend and which involve adults as stern teachers and taskmasters. The bush school, examined in Chapter 9, is one such institution that the Kpelle and other West African societies make use of. It transmits core values that reflect such fundamental aspects of adult character as proper gender relations, attitudes toward authority, and ideas about religion and mysticism.

We must not think of culture as some well-oiled machine, with cultural routines as buttons to be pushed at just the right point in a child's development. This is a loose, imperfect system. It is designed as much to minimize the investment in child rearing as it is to maximize the result. Chapter 10 discusses how the system seems to be breaking down in Gbarngasuakwelle. Also, we cannot conclude that all cultural routines—especially those practiced by parents—are necessarily efficacious. For example, from Riesman's (1992) study we learn that FulBe mothers frequently give their infants and small children enemas. Knowing that in West Africa, dehydration, brought on by parasite-induced diarrhea, is the major cause of child mortality in many areas, this practice is incredible. Here is a cultural routine designed to promote the health and well-being of children that, undoubtedly, has just the opposite effect.[15]

The notion that societies seek to minimize their investment in children—in direct contrast to our own child-centered outlook (Figure 2.1)—cannot be overstressed. Much child care is actually in the hands of one's slightly older brothers and sisters. The pervasiveness of "sib care" was first noted by Weisner and Gallimore (1977), who found, in a sample of more than 100 societies, that 40% of infants and 80% of toddlers are cared for primarily by someone other than their mother. Sutton-Smith (1977), in commenting on their study, notes:

> Maximal personal and social development of infants is produced by the mother (or caretaker) who interacts with them in a variety of stimulating and playful ways. Unfortunately the intelligence to do this with ever more exciting contingencies is simply not present in child caretakers. It is difficult enough to impart these ideas of infant stimulation even to mothers. As the review demonstrates so well, children as major caretakers maintain social life at a much lower level. (p. 184)

Rogoff (1990), in reviewing a controlled study on these young caretaker/teachers, concludes: "Most of the child teachers appeared insensitive to their partner's need to learn, providing little guidance and almost no preparation for the test" (p. 165). But, if we see the role of sib caretakers not as teachers in the way that mainstream parents are in the United States, but as models for their charges to imitate (Chapter 5) and as their guardians, they may fill these roles admirably (Zukow, 1989). Again, it is *our* society that seeks "*maximal* personal and social development. . . ." This is not the case elsewhere (see especially Harkness et al., 1992).

Just as children have multiple caretakers, so, too, there is a great deal of redundancy built in to a society's stock of culture routines, as the epigraph that began this chapter asserts. As we shall see, for example, Kpelle children are liberally showered with moralistic tales and proverbs that incorporate a limited store of themes. One such theme is embodied in the proverb, "What killed the chicken will be found in its gullet": Do not blame others for your own calamities.

SUMMARY

All societies must deal with the problem of rearing children to become fully human and competent practitioners of their own culture. Human children are, initially, quite helpless and they are far from being behavioral clones. Developmental psychology, heavily influenced by contemporary, mainstream European and American values, has seen the burden of this task as being borne by parents who actively and vigilantly "rear" their children (Damon, 1995). When we examine other societies, however, we see a different picture. Far from being the all-consuming task it appears to be in our society, parents spend relatively little time actively shaping their children's behavior either by word or deed. Caretaking is much more diffuse and incorporates the service of co-wives, grandparents, neighbors, siblings, and play groups. Each has a well-known role to play. Siblings, in particular, have much responsibility for child minding. Major milestones in the individual's development also serve to reprogram the behavior of the child and his or her significant others. In the village we also see more clearly the presence of routine enculturating media such as games, folktales, and apprenticeship that are stored in the minds of older individuals who model them for novices to imitate. People assume that children acquire their culture, primarily through observation and imitation rather than direct instruction. Hence, children are encouraged to hang around adults, to play under their watchful eyes on the mother-ground, and to try on adult practices in make-believe. Finally, we note that the public and routinized nature of these practices reinforces a conservative ethos. All these things are done by and for children because they are "proper."

Before focusing on the culture of children and the routines that prepare them for adulthood, we must first get a picture of what an adult's life and responsibilities are. What does it mean to say one is Kpelle? Chapter 3 provides an overview of Kpelle culture, as practiced in the interior Liberian village of Gbarngasuakwelle.

CHAPTER 3

The Research Setting

An examination of Kpelle culture reveals the tremendous respect
paid to tradition.

—GAY AND COLE (1967, p. 15)

The earliest travelers/anthropologists were expected to provide an ency-
clopedic inventory of customs, rituals, and economic practices—among
other things—for the "tribe" they had chosen to study. As these classic
ethnographies accumulated, it became possible, indeed desirable, to do
more focused ethnography. Anthropologists concerned themselves with a
more restricted area of culture, which would be studied in depth. The
Kpelle have been the subjects of several such focused studies.

KPELLE STUDIES

For example, in the late 1950s Jim Gibbs (1963, 1965/1988), working in
Panta Chiefdom, studied Kpelle law and judicial proceedings. A decade
later, Buddy Bellman (1975, 1983), working primarily in the village of Su-
cromo, immersed himself in the world of Kpelle sorcery and secret societies. A few years later, Catherine Bledsoe (1980), based in Fuama Chiefdom, conducted a thorough study of Kpelle marriage.

By the mid-1970s, funds for West African ethnography had become
scarcer—Thomasson's (1987) dissertation on Kpelle ironwork is one of
the few studies from that period. Then, in April 1980, Samuel Doe led a
group of army officers in overthrowing the presidency of William Tolbert
and, in the process, ending the 100+-year hegemony of the "Americo-
Liberians"—descendants of the freed slaves who had been returned to
Africa between 1822 and 1879. Tolbert's demise ushered in an era of instability in Liberia that continues to the present day and all but precludes
such activity by foreign academics as ethnographic study. In short, a sub-

stantial body of writing about the Kpelle people exists, but most of it is at least 20 years old.

At a population more than 200,000, the Kpelle represent the largest single tribe in Liberia. They inhabit the central region of the country as well as neighboring Guinea, where they are referred to as Guerzè. The Kpelle language was placed by Murdock (1959) in the Peripheral Mande category. In effect, they share much linguistically and culturally with other West African societies—notably the *Poro* and *Sande* secret society complex. The people now known as Kpelle migrated from the savannah south and west of the Sahara to their present home—forcing out their predecessors—around 1600 (Schultz, 1973). Aside from warfare related to territorial conquest, the Kpelle were at the center of intervillage and intertribal rivalry for control of lucrative trade routes—especially the trade in slaves. It was not until the mid-19th century that the abolition of slavery and the pacifying effects of the Americo Liberian colonists brought relative peace to the region (Bledsoe, 1980).

The Kpelle are an agrarian people whose lives revolve around upland or swidden rice cultivation. Marriage, household composition, and settlement patterns are dictated by the labor requirements of rice farming. Rice is both staple and the foundation of the economy, serving as a store of wealth and a medium of exchange. The goal of rice farming is not just to feed the population but to provide a sufficient surplus to afford a varied and complex culture. That is, efficient production of rice allows many Kpelle to devote their energies to other pursuits, notably such crafts as blacksmithing, woodworking, and weaving; medicines and sorcery; hunting and gathering; and animal husbandry.

Another factor that dominates Kpelle life is the "bush," primary and secondary forest and scrub that provides a cornucopia of useful products including game, delicacies, and medicines. The bush also affords a ready supply of characters to people the rich library of Kpelle stories, songs, and myths. This folklore, in turn, is a fundamental part of Kpelle enculturation, as we will see.

Gibbs (1963, p. 16) refers to the *Poro* as the "cement" of Kpelle society. This all-encompassing men's secret society is the "main coercive agent; psychologically and physically" (Fulton, 1972, p. 1221), as well as being the "earthly manifestation . . . of [Kpelle] religion" (p. 1227). Aside from a few political offices (e.g., town chief and paramount chief), men who seek power and prestige do so within the elaborately graded hierarchy of the *Poro* (Fulton, 1968, 1972). Its sister organization, the *Sande*, functions in similar fashion for women's affairs.

In pursuing my study of Kpelle childhood, I consulted at length with Americans who had lived among the Kpelle for many years, as well as with more acculturated Kpelle who had traveled in the Liberian interior. I wanted a research site that was relatively unacculturated, no school, church or store as yet; one that was relatively large with a concomitantly large population of children but that was, for medical reasons, at least, not wildly inaccessible. We settled on Gbarngasuakwelle, pronounced barn-ga-suuaah-k (plosive sound)-weh-leh.

GBARNGASUAKWELLE

I remember my first night in Gbarngasuakwelle as if it were yesterday. Although only 300 kilometers from the capital Monrovia, the trip by jitney, four-wheel-drive truck, and foot had taken more than 12 hours. I could barely stand long enough to pay my respects to Town Chief Wollokollie. Then, in the middle of the night, one of the worst malaria attacks I have ever had, awakened fears that my long and expensive journey would come to a premature conclusion.[1] Fortunately, within 3 days I was well enough to begin, with Paul Ricks, a survey of the town and to conduct a census of 6- to 13-year-olds.

Gbarngasuakwelle lies at 7.5° longitude by 9° latitude in the tropical rain forest belt that separates the African savannah from the West African coast. Situated about 4 miles from the Guinea border, the town occupies an area of about 5 hectares of level ground at the edge of an escarpment. The 160 houses are scattered almost at random, some far apart, others quite close together. "This was a strategic device in the past, when inhabitants tried to confuse invading enemies" (Bledsoe, 1980, p. 43).

There are four "quarters" (*kwilli*), one dominated by the town chief's house, the second by Firestone's house and shop, the third by Jawo Bonah's house, and the last by the Mandingos' mosque/shop building. Irregular-shaped open areas between houses serve as playgrounds (*panaŋ lè-ma* = mother-ground) and for court disputes (Plate 3.1). The construction of the houses varies: Some are round, some rectangular, some have thatched roofs, others corrugated iron roofs. Benches stand adjacent to houses, which front on the open areas. There are a few trees in the town and behind some houses are gardens. Small, cylinder-shaped buildings adjoin each house; these are kitchens. Surrounding the town on three sides is scrub brush and a few ancient trees and clusters of banana, papaya, and oil palm. One portion of the surrounding bush is high for-

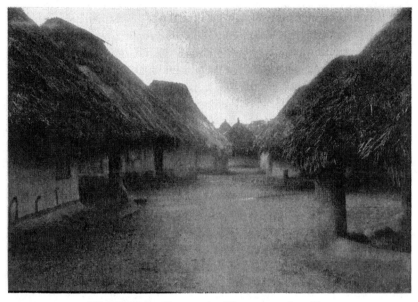

PLATE 3.1. Houses in Gbarngasuakwelle.

est. This area is fenced off from the town and is forbidden to all but *Poro* society members. Paths bisect the bush leading to farms, which surround the town. Streams and swampy areas dot the perimeter. The bush has been under cultivation for at least 100 years; hence, native flora and fauna have been reduced substantially.

There are two seasons: the rainy lasting from May to October, the dry from November to April. In the middle months of the dry season there will be no rain whatsoever, yet humidity will hover around 90%, and the temperature seldom falls below 30°. In the middle months of the rainy season, thunderstorms occur every day with precipitation of 2.5 centimeters or more per day.

The population of Gbarngasuakwelle is approximately 800, 90% of whom are Kpelle, the remaining 10% Mandingo. The latter speak a dialect of the Bambara language group, as well as some Kpelle and some English. They have migrated from the north and east into Liberia and are ubiquitous throughout the country as petty traders. In habit and custom they are quite different from the Kpelle majority.

The people all have a slender, well-muscled physique. Men wear robes or Western-style pullover shirts and short trousers. The women wrap a length of cloth (1.3 meters × 1 meter), a lappa in Liberian English, around their waist, and sometimes cover their hair with a head tie. Shoes are worn rarely by either sex. The principal adornment is cicatrized markings on the skin, put there when the person is initiated into the *Poro* or *Sande*. Women also wear silver or brass bracelets and multistrand necklaces made of tiny glass beads.

Life expectancy is low and infant mortality high due to the large array of endemic diseases and parasites. A few of the more common maladies include schiastosomiasis, malaria, ringworm, hookworm, leprosy, amoebic dysentery, typhus, and tuberculosis. Women begin bearing children at approximately age 17, and continue to do so, if physically able, at the rate of one birth every 3 years until they are near 40. Partly because of the high death rate, medicine, sorcery, and witchcraft are important elements of the culture.

Individuals' lives are governed by three interacting forces: tradition, ambition, and retribution. The ideal is tradition. People are expected to behave in a prescribed manner, to cultivate a rice farm, to build and maintain a house, to care for children, to join the *Poro* or *Sande* society, and to mind their own business. This is the minimum expected of a "citizen." If a person does these things and lives long, he or she gradually is elevated to a position of respect and will serve as a wise adviser to friends and offspring and aid in the governance of the town through participation in town councils and the courts. But there are also inducements to strive for more than this minimum. Polygyny is valued over monogamy. One should have a surplus of rice to avoid going into debt, at the same time, helping out less fortunate relatives. One can also strive for the prestige of a skilled job such as blacksmithing, the political position of town chief, or the politicoreligious position of *Zò*. All these positive traits seemed to be embodied in Wollokollie, the town chief and one of my principal informants. (I lived in a corner of his large and diversely populated house.)

There are two broad avenues to these goals, hard work and efficient management of one's resources and a reputation for fairness in dealing with others or sorcery, witchcraft, thievery, and exploitation of one's advantage over others. The latter course is expedient and dangerous, but most ambitious individuals use a combination of sanctioned and unsanctioned means to achieve power. However, overambition is checked through various forces of retribution. These are the moot and town chief's courts, which penalize the overly ambitious through fines and public ridicule. The power of secret societies and *Zò-na* ("medicine persons") exacts swift and often deadly punishment. Finally, the force of public opinion is vented through gossip and other forms of harassment to keep an individual in check.

FOREST AND TOWN

The Kpelle world is divided into two main categories: forest things and town things (Cole et al., 1971). Both locations have good and bad qualities. The forest is where farms and gardens are planted and where hunting and trapping take place and thus is associated with sustenance. But the forest also houses evil things such as genii, water spirits, and witches. In town one has one's house, family, and friends gathered around, but strangers including *Kwii* people can find someone more easily in the town and make trouble, by expropriating the person's property or making *kpamo* (sorcery) against the person.

Perhaps the most salient town–forest distinction is that between town work and forest work. There is "talking matter" or dispute settlement, especially the town chief's court and the moot (a gathering of the elders associated with a particular household), which takes place in town. Other town work includes "fixing up the town" and "building things," which everyone engages in, and skilled work such as blacksmithing, leatherwork, and wood carving, which are done by specialists.

The major category of forest work is rice farming, which is the paramount work class. The rice is an upland variety and the planting technique is to clear an area of brush, burn it, then sow the seed among the remaining tree stumps. The various tasks of the rice cycle are broken down into categories and assigned to specific groups; that is, tree felling is done by men, planting by women, and chasing birds away from the ripening crop by boys. Several of these categories are done by *kuus*, which are cooperative work parties. *Kuu* membership cuts across household lines and each member of the *kuu* is allotted a full day's work on his or her farm by the entire *kuu*. Two percussionists may accompany the *kuu* as it is working and then, at the end of the day, play as the workers dance and sing to celebrate their accomplishments.

Rice is used both as the staple food and as a means of savings. It is stored in cylindrical kitchens built near the farm site. It is taken out and milled to prepare a meal or to trade for other needed goods. Each member of the household over age 12 will be allotted a share of the harvest to use as he or she sees fit. The bulk of the harvest is kept by the household head to meet his own and the household's needs.

Other crops are planted as well. Women plant cassava, peppers, and a variety of "greens"; men take care of oil palm trees, pissava palms (for palm wine), cocoa, banana, and coffee trees. The forest is also a source of wild game, including fish in the streams which are caught by a variety of traps (men) or nets (women), land snails, several varieties of deer men hunt for singly or in large groups, and birds, which are trapped or shot down with a sling.

Medicine bridges the town and the forest. Leaves, roots, bark, and so on needed in preparing medicines must be found in the forest. The medicines are made and used in the town. Much medicine knowledge is shared only among members of various secret societies, such as the snake (*Kalisali*) society, whose members specialize in curing poisonous snake bites. These societies are voluntary associations, but nearly every adult belongs to at least one of them. The *Poro* and *Sande* are said to be the "father" and "mother" of the secret societies. A man or woman who has mastered many medicines and risen to the top in several secret societies may apply the title of *Zò* to him- or herself. These people fulfill key authority roles in the *Sande* and *Poro* as well as being curers.

HOUSEHOLD, FAMILY, AND CHILDREN

The household is the basic kin, economic, and political unit of the town. The household may consist of more than one actual house, but there will be only one household head, usually a male. The household is held together primarily by shared work (Plate 3.2). Members of the same household work together to maintain the house and the farm and share the proceeds of their labor. All the younger members of the household refer to the head as father regardless of blood relationship and the head's first wife as mother. The head nominally owns a parcel of land and he exercises control over where each member will make his or her rice farm, where he or she will sleep, who the unmarried females of the household will marry and so on. Bledsoe (1980) refers to "wealth-in-people." (p. 48). "Wealth and social standing rest, not on the amount of land a person owns . . . but rather on the number of people he or she can muster for farm work . . ." (p. 52). "Kpelle stratification is based primarily on the production of economic surpluses to attract dependents" (p. 48).

Disputes among household members are abhorrent and every attempt is made to settle them privately. If this is not possible, a moot is convened and if the elders in the moot are unable to restore harmony, at least

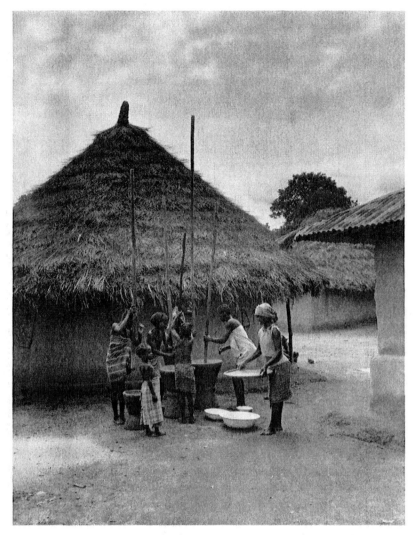

PLATE 3.2. Family work party.

one of the disputing parties will be forced out of the household. The larger and more harmonious a household, the greater prestige that accrues to
the head. By the same token, orphans, widows, unmarried males, and otherwise unattached individuals gravitate to the household of a man with
high prestige, confident of his care and protection. In any interhousehold
dispute, the head can count on the allegiance of all those presently and
formerly members of his household.

There are a number of alternative procedures for arranging a marriage, but the man must pay a brideprice in goods or service to his wife's father. Once married, the wife incurs three responsibilities to her husband: bearing and raising children, working on his farm, and taking care of his demands for food and sex. "Women work almost continuously on rice farms. Their main tasks, planting, weeding and harvesting, are long and arduous. . . . Though women spend more time farming than men, they also spend more time on such auxiliary activities as making oil, growing vegetables, catching fish, . . . and they assume the greatest responsibility for feeding the family" (Bledsoe, 1980, pp. 31–32). Children are valued for their labor on the farm, male offspring are expected to care for aging parents, and females bring in bride-wealth or bride-service.

Men play no role in the birth of their offspring. The mother is aided by her mother, sisters, and a midwife. As long as she is nursing the child, usually until it is 2½ years old, her husband may not have intercourse with her and if she is one of several co-wives, his other demands will lessen as well. The infant sleeps with the mother and is carried on her back. It will be fed on demand, and this signals a general attitude of permissiveness with respect to infants and toddlers.

Girls begin helping their mothers with such chores as carrying water and helping with a younger sibling by age 5. Boys are free to play until the age 7 or 8, when their fathers begin to take them along on hunting and trapping expeditions and give them their first machete for cutting brush. The children under 8 in a household form a tightly knit play group and engage together in various types of make-believe play. Older girls in a household also form play groups for such games as *Nyinaŋ* and dancing. Boys have considerably more freedom to form play groups that cut across household lines. They play a number of games and gather at night to tell stories.

Gradually, the household's expectations for the child escalate and he or she must now begin carrying out designated chores for the family on a regular basis. Failure to do so results in verbal abuse and beating. Children also gradually acquire certain skills such as making fishnet, spinning thread, weaving mats, making traps, building a house, and so on, from their parents or older siblings. More important than any particular skill, however, are two attitudes children must develop: (1) working hard without complaint, and (2) showing respect and deference to anyone older than themselves.

Bush school is a major event in the lives of children of both sexes. Little is known about it with certainty because it is closed to outsiders, but all girls and all boys must join the *Sande* and *Poro* societies, respectively. It is a frightening experience for them as they are taken from the comfort and safety of their homes into the forest, terrorized by masked figures, and cicatrized by *Ƶò-na*. The total effect is to produce a lasting respect and fear of the secret societies and medicines. The return from bush school signals a change in the child's status in the household, which is signaled by by the new, permanent names given them by the *Ƶò-na*. Only in late adolescence, however, do individuals begin to join voluntary secret societies and learn to make and use medicines.

As indicated earlier, a prime avenue toward higher status for a man is to have a large and harmonious household. Marrying several wives may accomplish this, but only if the wives are fertile and take good care of the children. Barrenness and miscarriages are common and lead to acrimonious disputes, which end in divorce. If an apparently healthy child dies, its mother is immediately suspected of having been neglectful. For example, if a mother drops her baby accidentally, anyone who sees this will immediately run and beat her and she must submit, without resistance, to the beating. On the other hand, a mother who loses a child will almost automatically accuse a co-wife, or her husband's sister, of having "eaten" the child (as a witch) because of jealousy. Thus barren women suffer the dual agony of not having any offspring plus the frequent accusation that their jealousy has caused them to kill the children of related women.

A larger household has two advantages over a smaller one. The more individuals there are, the lighter will be the burden of work on any single individual. For example, in a large household the chore of cooking may be shared among four co-wives and several adolescent girls. Second, people prefer to work in groups, and in a large household nearly every task is conducted by a group rather than a single individual. Group members can converse, sing, and joke as they work. Members of any household must balance the traditional demands of rice farming and maintaining a house against the desire to enjoy themselves, to play. In a larger household there is both more free time for play and a greater likelihood that playful elements can be incorporated into the work.

When the Kpelle talk about their aspirations for their children, about their becoming competent adults, the ability *and desire* to acquire the skills associated with *tii*, or work, are paramount. It follows then that many cultural routines for children's development should point to one or more of these skills. In the next chapter, I offer an overview of the role of the Kpelle adult, focusing on the most important aspect of that role—*tii*.

CHAPTER 4

Kpelle Work

Do you expect to dig a rat hole and catch a deer in it?
—KPELLE PROVERB

The Kpelle define the ultimate end of their customary means of raising children as the production of a worker who lives in harmony with his or her fellows. This means that children must learn to work hard without complaint, to work cooperatively, and to master the specific skills that Kpelle work demands. As the proverb suggests, hard work is the highest virtue, a slacker the lowest of the low. Think for a moment about the process of focusing a camera lens. In the picture I want to capture in this book, children are in the foreground. But, in order to understand the end point of development—where children are heading—we must initially focus on the background, the life, and the work of adults. This chapter offers, then, a selective ethnography of the Kpelle—one that highlights *tii*, or work. As we shall see in subsequent chapters, this busy scene with a fore- and background is quite literal as well. Children are expected to hang around adults as they are working, to stand ready to help as needed, and, most important, to observe and imitate their behavior.

As an ethnographer, I acted as a naive observer, a novice, even a child. Once my purposes were clear, I was invited *everywhere* to witness for myself how the Kpelle build and maintain their society. However, no one ever volunteered to explain anything to me.[1] Although asking direct questions is considered bad manners at best, a form of sorcery at worst, I did not have 6 to 8 years to figure everything out by observation—as would be expected of a child or a woman who married in to the village. My informants understood that and were usually indulgent in answering my questions. None of the topics I pursued yielded as positive and supportive a response as my queries about the nature of *tii*. By contrast, medicine and sorcery were off limits, governed by *ifa mo* ("don't talk"). Similarly, child rearing was not fruitful because it is taken largely for granted and seen as of little consequence. But work was something everyone did, was proud of, and considered quintessentially Kpelle. In the rich store of Kpelle proverbs, there is an especially rich subgenre directed at the lazy and incompetent.

I began by trying to discover what activities the residents themselves considered to be work and how these were interrelated. The most straightforward procedure was to elicit a taxonomy of activities labeled *tii*. The taxonomy of work is a folk taxonomy. This means that rather than being created by a single individual or derived from a single set of facts or assumptions about nature, it has evolved and changed as the town and its inhabitants have changed. It is a taxonomy created by many people at many points in time so that no two informants will agree entirely on its construction. Broad distinctions such as that between town and forest are salient to these people, but in other areas, clear-cut distinctions were harder to arrive at and the logical bases of classes difficult to elucidate. For this reason it was necessary to draw on several sources in creating a taxonomy. Observation was helpful: it allowed me to make up a list of activities I, at least, called work, Later this list would be modified through structured questioning, such as "Is *X* work?" "What kind of work is *X*?" "Who does *X*?" "When is *X* done?" and so on. Still further modification was achieved through less structured interviews, especially with groups of men with whom debate would arise and eventually be resolved. For example, it was not until late in the questioning that the distinction between *Bare-tεε* (trapping animals) and *Sia loi kεε* (attacking animals) came out. It was a valid distinction in that everyone agreed on what would or would not belong to one or the other of these two classes, but it was not a distinction that is frequently made in talking about or doing hunting and the defining characteristics were vague (the complete taxonomy can be found in Lancy, 1975a).

Level I is, of course, work. Level II, town work and forest work, is the major division. A taxonomy of *sεŋ* (things), collected earlier for the Kpelle, similarly had town–forest as the major division (Cole et al., 1971, pp. 61–69). Level III includes some rather poorly defined and shifting class names, which are still quite general. The activities under the class name Buŋwoi-ti (lit., "walking in the bush") and the activities under *Sia-loi* (making farm) contrast sharply, but *Sia-loi* is not always recognized as the class name for these activities. Level IV includes "realms of work" which are clearly bounded but which either contain further subclasses, as in *Bare-tεε* (trapping), or are composed of many different activities such as *Koli-ɣale* (blacksmithing). There are 38 distinct level IV "genera." Level V items are specific work activities; they are minimal taxa which cannot be further broken down. There are, approximately, 80 of these species-level items, ranging from *Ya-kpɛ* (net fishing) to *Kpeliŋ-saa* (stool carving).

However, although this analysis of *tii* was thorough, the broader distinctions that people make when they talk about or do work are more relevant in the study of children's enculturation. Rice farming is both the paramount work activity and a focus for much of the village's activities. Everyone participates in some aspect of the rice cycle, including very young children. A great deal of medicine owes its symbolic power to its connection to the rice farm, such as the use during rituals of the hoe and other farm implements made by the blacksmith. Many court disputes arise over the allocation of land for planting rice, over the distribution of the rice harvest, and over the fair treatment of *kuu* members working on a rice farm. Nearly all other work activities must take place only after the tasks associated with rice farming are attended to. This includes hunting, trapping, tree planting, and so on. Materials to build a house, carved items, cloth, and medicines are usually acquired by trading with surplus rice.

If rice farming is the foundation on which the society rests, the courts, divining, ordeals and the secret societies all function to ensure social control and, in the absence of a strong central authority or code of laws, are crucial for maintaining peace and harmony. No trespass is treated lightly, from the sudden death of a young girl to adultery to the "borrowing" of a lantern. Each action must be accounted for and retribution must be exacted. Whether this accounting and retribution take place in the public arena of the courts or the private arena of secret medicines depends on the gravity of the offense and the extent to which premeditation and willful behavior is involved. The more serious the offense, the more likely it is to be handled secretly. The chief and the elders exercise their authority over transgressors by virtue of the respect they have earned and through the use of various dramatic "speech events." The *Ƶò-na*, diviners, and "devils" exercise their authority by virtue of the fear they arouse for their powers and through the use of various medicines. Children are not active participants in these events, but they are keen observers and may become the focal point of adult disputes—jealous co-wives, annoyed neighbors, paternity contestants.

Everyone is expected to do his or her part in rice farming, marketing, town cleanup, and so on, but there are optional tasks grouped under skilled work. Some skilled work is rudimentary and no special status is associated with its mastery. In general, there is an inverse relationship between the complexity of a skill and the number of people in town who have mastered it. Many tasks are done only by persons of a certain age and sex. A boy weaving a mat or a girl braiding a belt attracts no notice, but a boy weaving a bag or girl weaving a hammock will.

The remainder of this chapter describes the various classes of work included in the taxonomy. Emphasis is given to the kinds of things an individual must know in order to perform a given task. Thus, complex tasks are broken down into parts or steps, indicating the combination of skills (intellectual, sensorimotor, social) that the task appears to call for. Because weaving is so complex, for example, its description is much lengthier than that for, say, palm work. Also, tasks that appeared to demand high skill levels for successful performance, such as talking matter and medicine making, both rather demanding socially and intellectually, are given considerably more attention than cleaning up the town, which is less demanding.

MAKING A RICE FARM

In Gbarngasuakwelle work is *tii*, and *tii*, if left unqualified in general conversation, means rice farming. There are a variety of activities that can be classified *tii*, but all are secondary to rice farming. The assistant town chief, Nyanni, was ill and had not eaten anything for 2 days, but his expression was, "I haven't eaten rice for two days." By the same token, everyone who is physically able "makes rice farm," regardless of other work they may do, including individuals who are employed in the modern sector, such as the rubber tapper, the taxi driver, and the tailor, who could buy all the rice they needed to live on. I was subjected to this attitude, stressing the overriding importance of rice farming, almost daily. After I had made clear my intention to study traditional customs, my first guided tours were of rice farms. Later, when I concentrated on skilled work, which is done in the town, I was asked, incredulously, at the end of the day, "What, you mean you spent the whole day in town again?" Another typical interview went something like this:

"When are you going to start making a farm [rice]?"

"I'm not going to make a farm."

"Oh, you made one at home [in the United States] before you came?"

"No."

"Your wife is making it for you?"

"No."

"Your parents?"

"No."

"Your brothers and sisters?"

"No."

"But, how will you live?"

Rice as staple and symbol is ever present. In court cases one of the more common types of disputes centers on the allocation of land for rice farming or on the equitable distribution of the rice harvest. Boys and girls who are "reborn" as they leave the bush school are clothed in hats and skirts made of dried rice leaves. Rice is used as a savings account; when a woman or man needs some manufactured item such as a bolt of cloth, he or she will take out just enough rice from storage, beat it, clean it, then sell it by the cup to make the purchase. In folktales, by far the most commonly depicted work activity is rice farming.

Part of the reason for the focal importance of rice lies in the fact that its cultivation is so neatly cyclical. There is virtually no time during the year when some important operation connected with the rice farm is not going on. In late December and January the farmer picks out the area where he will plant next year's crop. He clears a small section of bush, about 0.5 meters square, which acts as a sign to others that the land is taken. Alternatively, a man may block off a path leading into a certain area as a sign that he intends to farm there.

Land is nominally "owned" by the paramount chief, or in earlier times by the town chief. In reality it is owned by lineage heads and passes from father to eldest son. Many individuals may make claims to parts of this land. A man's younger brothers, his unmarried or widowed daughters, his older sons, and his deceased brothers' wives all make requests for land from him. He, in turn, designates a general area much larger than necessary for a single farm, and individuals choose the best plot in this area. Kpelle residence is patrilocal, but I recorded cases of a son-in-law farming on his father-in-law's land. All who receive a share of land are expected to pay some token to the lineage head. This is not a fixed rent but depends on the user's financial circumstances and on his or her respect for the lineage head. The term "respect" deserves some explanation.

A young man or woman or an older "stranger" is greatly dependent on the older, influential townspeople. In the allocation of land for farming and for building a house, in dispute settlement, in the moot, in marriage, in the *Poro*, and in medicine making, the elders make decisions that are crucial in the lives of those younger than themselves. They expect and demand respect. This goes beyond the social interaction plane of using polite terms and gestures[2] and includes making small periodic gifts to "our fathers and mothers." Therefore, a younger person cannot settle any obligations he or she may have to an elder by a fixed periodic or large, lump-sum payment. When an individual uses the land of the lineage head, he or she is expected to make frequent gifts of produce and to perform chores on the lineage head's farm.

A number of factors are considered in the choice of a farm site. The most important is the length of time the area has lain fallow. The rice cycle runs a full year and a plot is cultivated only once; then the bush is allowed to take over the land for a period of 5 to 10 years. Experienced farmers can tell by the thickness of the tree trunks how long a given piece of land has been idle. If they have been farming the same general area for a long time, they will have stored in memory, like a string of knots on a cord, the locations of past farms. When we asked people the ages of their children they frequently began citing farm locations from the most recent location backwards until they came to the one that coincided with the birth of a child. By keeping a tally on their fingers they were able to accurately estimate the age.

The land should be as level as possible, which may not be very level considering the hilly terrain, and free of swamps. Distance from the town is another important factor. The further one goes from the town the more one finds little used and, hence, more fertile land. But there are drawbacks. Trees that have grown longer will have thicker trunks and be much harder to fell. The time and energy expended in getting to and from the farm may detract significantly from farmwork. Thus, many people establish second residences on these outlying farms and live there during peak work seasons. "Friendship" is often cited in the decision-making process. Individuals make every attempt to site their farms adjacent to friends. The term "friend" cuts across family lines. That is, an individual can have friends who may or may not also be members of his or her family. In getting to their farm, individuals must pass through other farms, and it is considered best to avoid contacts with those with whom they are not on friendly terms. On the positive side, friends on adjacent farms will often help each other with tasks that do not require a full *kuu*. Also, the treks to and from the farm each day are important occasions for conversation, and a large group of friends heading off to neighboring farms makes for a lively party. Finally, there are intangibles which can be covered by the term "luck." Certain sites are considered unlucky because they have failed to yield much rice in the past, because a serious accident occurred there, or because the diviner has indicated the site is unlucky. Other unlucky sites are those over which disputes arose about the division of the harvest.

Choosing a farm site, then, is not a "snap" process. Traveling to and from this year's farm, the owner passes through the bush that may contain next year's farm and all its associated memories. Long before the time comes to mark off next year's plot, he will have decided on a general area, or on several likely alternatives.

Once the plots have been allocated and chosen, the land is "owned" by those who farm it. The lineage head's widowed sister-in-law, for example, owns the particular plot of land she has chosen for the duration of the season. She arranges for the formation of cooperative work parties (*kuu*) and determines when a particular phase of the farming cycle will begin. The first phase is cutting the thick underbrush. This is done by a *kuu* composed of men and women between 12 and 40 years of age. Working in a line with their backs to the brush, they cut with machetes in an arc. As the brush is cut it is folded down by pressure from their backs and legs and then trampled under foot. Those who are less able to stand the strain of this demanding task follow behind and gather the cut brush into piles.

In late March, a second *kuu*, this time composed of men only, cuts down trees that were left standing after the first cutting. Kola, cottonwood (Kapok), pissava, and palm trees are left standing. Trees are cut off at about 3 feet above the ground and are left to rot or dry where they fall. Branches are cut off and these are piled with the dry brush. Each of these *kuus* has a leader and usually a second in command. The leader is responsible for forming the *kuu* and letting it know when and where it is to work. The whole *kuu* labors on each *kuu* member's farm in rotation and *kuus* may not break up for many years. The *kuu* leader is usually a person in his or her physical prime, someone who is not frequently sick and can work regularly. He or she contacts friends and/or relatives and forms the *kuu*. The second in command arranges for the distribution of food, which the "owner" is expected to provide. The person whose turn it is to have the *kuu* on his or her farm owns the *kuu* for that day and may make stipulations about what and how much work is to be done. Disputes often arise because an owner has asked for too much work or provided too little food, and members of the *kuu* may refuse to work on that person's farm the next time around. On the other hand, a *kuu* member who is often absent or late, or a slack worker will be fined or otherwise penalized. Again, respect is a factor; a *kuu* owner or member will often be accused of lacking respect for the other members. Because upland rice is the staple crop and no labor-saving technology or draft animals exist, the *kuu* is vital to survival. There is little leeway in Gbarngasuakwelle for the individualist, the eccentric, the recluse who wants to "go it alone." Households are never large enough to manage the farmwork without occasional outside help. No household head is so powerful that he can force his family members to work against their will.

After the brush has dried sufficiently, it is fired and the ash constitutes the only source of fertilizer for the crop. When to fire the farm is a touchy decision, and a farmer may resort to a diviner to guide him. If he does it too early the dead growth may not be sufficiently dry to sustain a good fire. If he waits too long the rain, which begins in May, will soak everything. After burning, the farmer and his sons or brothers take the unburned trunks and stack them to one side of the field. These will be used for firewood and, if not badly charred, for house poles. Planting is done from late May to September, periods when the rainfall lessens. Girls and women form a *kuu* to cut the brush that has grown up in the interim since burning and to loosen the soil with short-handled hoes (Plate 4.1). They, too, work in a line with their backs to the unworked soil, bending from the waist. One woman, often the *kuu* "owner," scatters seed rice from a pan over the area that has been prepared. Men are busy fencing in the fields to keep out groundhogs and making storage huts, called kitchens in Liberia.

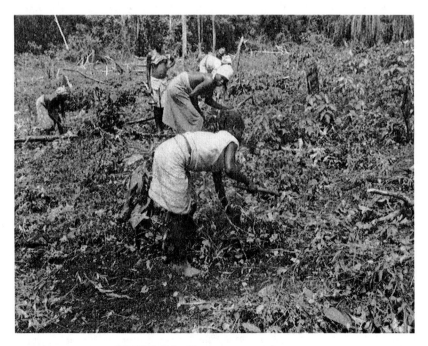

PLATE 4.1. Young women hoeing.

The rice kitchens are cylindrical with conical thatched roofs. The inside of the thatched portion is the rice loft and has a trapdoor underneath. The structure is supported on thick posts and is usually unwalled. In the center of the kitchen is the fire for cooking and drying meat, which hangs over it in a cage-like dryer.

The hard work of rice farming is now finished and a period of tension and anxiety sets in. If the previous year's crop was bad, rice stocks are low and Liberians speak of it being "hungry time." Two things are crucial at this stage, the rain and the birds. Ideally, the rice should have regular showers for about 3 months, but too much rain or too hard a rain will damage the crop. I recorded at least six species of birds which feed on the rice crop. Some travel in huge flocks with a thousand members. They perch in the trees that have been left standing in the fields and at the first opportunity swoop down to devour a crop. Young boys are assigned the vital task of chasing away birds. They do this by pounding on sticks and by well-placed shots from their slingshots. When the rice gets full, everyone joins in the bird-chasing task. The importance of attending to the rice cycle and to one's neighbor's crop becomes paramount. If all the rice ripens at approximately the same time, no single farm suffers too badly from the birds because they are spread out, but if an individual's crop should ripen well before or well after that of his or her neighbors, the birds will clean the individual out. Continuous attention must also be paid to weeds and groundhogs. Fortunately, the rice appears to be disease and insect resistant.

Harvesting is done by men and women in *kuus* in late October to December. Harvesters hold a small knife in one hand and several stalks are bunched together in the other hand and then cut them off at the base. The stalks are first piled on a scaffold to dry, then carried into the loft. The stalks are removed from the loft in anticipation of a meal, They are placed in a large mortar and beaten with a heavy pestle. The grains, being heavier, fall to the bottom of the depression, which is funnel-shaped. The bare stalks are then thrown out or may later be used as ticking. A smaller mortar and pestle are used in separating the kernels from the husks. Together they are poured into a woven tray with sloping sides called, in Liberian English, a fanner. The fanner is shaken back and forth, then flipped abruptly as the person backs away so that the husks fly out onto the ground. Further cleaning is done by hand to remove stones and chaff. The rice is cooked in water in large cast-iron pots over a fire.

After the harvest there is a relaxed period culminating in a celebration which, strangely, falls on Christmas Day. The end of the cycle falls in

December to January and the principal task is to divide the rice. A portion will be allocated as seed rice for next season. A second portion will be set aside to be sold to pay the government hut tax, which comes due in January. The head of the household must also divide a portion among his wives and older children and among other individuals who were living under his roof and helping in the farm during the year. Sometimes this decision is accomplished in the field. That is, after the farm is laid out, the farmer subdivides it and designates areas that now belong to each of his wives and to his children who are over 14 but not yet on their own, For the entire season all these minifarms will be worked as one large farm, but, at harvest time, each will be harvested separately with each individual owner keeping the produce from his or her minifarm. In fact, in laying out the farm, the household head may well walk off sections, the produce of which he will later allocate, and in this way arrive at a reasonable size projected to meet his household's needs. There is no particular value attached to growing a large surplus.

Although villagers view rice as essential to their existence, outsiders quickly realize that other forms of work are equally significant in guaranteeing survival. The blacksmith is accorded high status because he makes the tools to work the farm, but other skilled workers make equally essential items. Hunting and fishing are treated as casual labor, yet they supply necessary and otherwise unavailable protein. One can eat rice without "soup" but not soup without rice, but the greens and vegetables that make up the soup supply essential vitamins. In the sections that follow, I show how work classes are grouped and the nature of work besides rice farming.

BUSH WORK

I was unable to obtain an aerial view of Gbarngasuakwelle, but if I had I would have seen something closely resembling a wagon wheel in shape. The town itself is the hub and radiating out from it are spokes. Each spoke, sometimes several adjacent spokes, belongs to one family or head of household, and each is divided into clearly delineated zones.

At the edge of the town are huge tall trees, left from the days when the whole town was ringed with trees and battlements to protect the inhabitants from raiding parties from other towns. Around these trees are the small vegetable gardens, usually tended by women, who grow tomatoes, cabbage, okra, eggplant, collard greens and bitterball. Further out on the spoke are plantings of bananas, papaya, cocoa, coffee, oranges, and sugar cane. These plants ripen at odd times; thus, they are strategically placed along paths leading to the rice farms so that the family will not miss the fruits. Joining this area, but further out, are patches planted with peanuts, cassava, and peppers, which, in turn, border the rice farm. These crops are secondary to the rice, but peanuts and cassava are both planted extensively and act as supplements to the steady rice diet. Hot peppers season every meal. Corn, cotton, and palms dot the rice farm itself. Most of the crops have been introduced within the last 100 years. This is certainly true of rubber, sugar cane, cocoa, and coffee, which are grown as cash crops. There is no particular ritual or honor associated with planting them. As I have stressed, rice is *the* crop. At the end of the spoke is unfarmed or rarely farmed country that is ideally suited to hunting. The largest of these zones is the land devoted to rice cultivation. At one time, no doubt, the forest was predominant, but Gbarngasuakwelle is ringed with other towns, all of which appear to be growing and all encroaching on her wheel rim. Hunters speak of the decline of game, especially the larger species such as elephant and buffalo.

"Walking about in the bush" is only provisionally a category of work. Hunting and trapping are viewed almost as they are by Americans (i.e., as a sport). Hunting and trapping of groundhogs, rats, monkeys, and certain birds is, however, work, in as much as these animals menace the rice crops. Taking other types of game, especially deer, also becomes work when either there is a failure of the rice harvest and hunger threatens or when the hunter is in need of quick cash which can be raised from the sale of meat.

In group hunting, men and boys are called together by a farmer who has noticed the tracks of large game in the forest adjacent to his farm. The group fans out in a rough circle around the area and begins advancing forward, tightening the circle like the drawstring on a sack, until the animal is located. Then all pounce at once. In net hunting one group fans out in a semicircle holding nets between them to block the animal's escape while the other group drives the animal toward the nets by shouting, clapping and beating sticks together.

Children "hunt" for snails. Snails are found under piles of rotting vegetation and are, of course, perfectly camouflaged. Finding them in the semidarkness that prevails in the bush takes practice. (I went on an outing with three young friends. The score for the afternoon: group = 60 snails, Lancy = 2 snails.)

There are many types of trapping. Some traps are made in town and are town work; others are made on the spot. Small streams bisect the country around Gbarngasuakwelle and these harbor crawfish and at least four species of fish. *Bunuŋ* is one type of woven fish trap that is baited and left in the water overnight. It is bullet-shaped and the rounded end is open. Inside is an inverted cone made like a fishnet with a small opening. Once the fish swims in, he has nearly an impossible time trying to get out. A stream may be dammed with a fence of sticks lashed with vines and, as fish collect at the fence, they are scooped up by hand. Another type of fence trap is a semicircle attached to the bank. Bait is floated on the water inside the trap and a patient fisherman releases a trapdoor once a fish has swum inside, then throws medicine in the water to stun the fish.

There are a variety of *gwala-tee*, or snare traps, which vary in size according to the animal that is anticipated. A trapper picks up the animal's spoor and knows from experience what kind it is. He looks especially for a path the animal seems to have worn and places his snare along this path. All snares are powered by a bent sapling and may be triggered by and catch the animal's foot or neck. *Bare-kuli* is the most elaborate of all traps. It is a fence woven of palm leaves and stands about 3.5 meters high and runs through the bush for as much as 100 meters. Every 5 meters is a square opening at the bottom of the fence and, on the far side away from the game, a snare, so that as the animal negotiates along the fence and discovers a hole, it puts its head through and releases the snare.

The rice farm and the oil palm are closely interlinked. A bowl of rice will, at the least, have a sauce of oil made by pounding in the mortar the palm kernel, or endocarp of the palm fruit. Furthermore, the oil palm, of all trees, is invariably left standing when land is cleared for a farm, and as the women clean and weed the rice farm, the men are often found nearby doing *tou-tii*. The oil palm has two strikingly different manifestations. As an immature tree with a height of up to 10 meters it looks squat and the crown of branches points upward. At maturity it reaches, slim and graceful, to a crown of over 30 meters and now the branches arch out and down from the crown. The immature tree is climbed via a log that has had notches cut out for footholds and a fork at the end to catch the trunk of the palm just below the crown. Adolescent boys of 10 and up can master the difficult task of climbing this precarious ladder and then, with a long-handled knife, cuting loose the cluster of palm fruits. The mature tree is climbed by men who walk up the trunk supported by a *Baliŋ* which encircles the trunk and goes around the back and is gripped by both hands on either side. The *Baliŋ* is made of vines and fibers lashed together and resembles an oval-shaped hula hoop. From his belt, the climber ties the long-handled knife and a machete to clear away dead branches.

The outer covering, or pericarp, of the fruit is beaten in the mortar and the yellowish paste is then mixed with water and potash to make soap. The kernels are either bagged and sold or beaten into palm oil. Another palm (pissava in Liberian English) is smaller and has no edible fruits, but its sap, which ferments in a cavity at the crown of the tree, is drunk as palm wine, which is the staple drink. The pissava palm is climbed with the ladder and a short-handled, long-bladed knife is used to gouge and hack an opening in the sap cavity which begins to leak its contents into a pail attached to the tree. The principal skill here is in knowing when to tap the tree; too early and the sap is sugary, too late and it is overripe and tastes rank. The wine is cleaned of dirt and debris, then decanted into a large round gourd to transport to the town. Approximately 50 to 75% of the palm wine brought into town in the evening is sold by the owners and the cries of "Come, let's drink" (i.e., come buy palm wine) can be heard in every quarter.

TOWN WORK

Talking Matter and Making Market

There is an open-air, transparent quality to Kpelle work and children can aquire much of the "basics" through observation. This quality made the work of the ethnographer all the more difficult as people found it hard to describe and explain the obvious. Talking matter (dispute settlement) proved to be the most challenging work category to study. It seemed to be quite important because such a large proportion of the men's time was taken up by it. Also, the most prosperous and influential men in town were the principal participants as town chief, assistant town chief, and elders. Yet, unlike other areas of work, the actual tasks performed by these men were far from obvious. A description of several cases would not have been sufficient to show what these men do in the course of talking matter. Hence, an analysis of talking matter based on many court observations was necessary. As I have described this analysis at length elsewhere (Lancy, 1980c), I offer only a brief summary here.

Nearly every Kpelle male, at some time in his life, will be a court participant. Gibbs (1963), for example, found that 85% of the Kpelle males in his survey acknowledged their involvement on one or more occasions in an adultery proceeding. The most important task for the litigant is to command several unnamed but highly stylized forms of elocution or speech events. I have labeled these the self-evident, staged anger, penitent, rhetorical questioning, and "reasonable man" speeches. Of course, proverbs figure heavily in court discourse as well. Each of these speech events has a characteristic tone and vocabulary and is used at different points in the proceedings. For example, once a decision appears to have gone against an individual, it is appropriate for the individual to shift into the penitent mode to lessen the severity of the fine. One effective (in my opinion) penitent speaker was given a stiff fine anyway because (according to the chief) he had waited too long to shift into the penitent speech mode.

Most of the cases I recorded were from the *koti-meni-saa*, or town chief's court (Plate 4.2). But there are other types of hearings, such as the *poloŋ-meni-saa*—house matter or moot. Procedures vary, of course, but the skills required of a successful plaintiff–defendant are similar. I should note that there is no onus in Kpelle society in being involved in legal matters per se unless one makes a habit of it. The importance of the court cannot be overestimated in terms of the maintenance of order in Gbarngasuakwelle. There are no police in the town; the *Poro* functions to control certain kinds of transgressions, but the vast majority of dis-

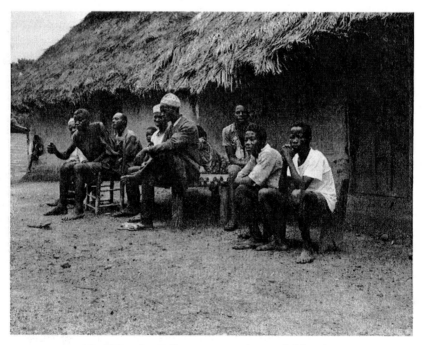

PLATE 4.2. Talking matter (note children).

putes that arise are beyond its "jurisdiction." The Kpelle traditionally have not had a strong centralized government, nor is the family and clan structure effective as a means to achieve social control. In examining the etiology of many disputes I was struck by the fact that the first step taken by one or the other of the disputants was often to at least threaten to sue the other party in court.

Men, women, and children are involved in marketing, but each in a somewhat different way. In Gbarngasuakwelle, as in other Kpelle towns, trading in large quantities of produce and selling imported items are almost entirely in the hands of the Mandingo people. An exception in Gbarngasuakwelle is Firestone, who runs a shop and is quite prosperous. He was, however, born and raised in Guinea, where trading is more widespread among the Kpelle. Otherwise, no one in Gbarngasuakwelle maintains a permanent shop, nor is there a communitywide market or market day, but everyone sells something at some time. Such perishable items as meat and vegetables are sold immediately, but such nonperishable items as rice and woven and carved things are made or prepared only when the person needs money for a purchase.

Rice, in 100-pound bags, palm kernels, unshelled peanuts, cocoa/coffee, and Kola nuts are sold by men to Mandingo or Lebanese traders and here the buyer sets the price per pound. Sellers are easily cheated because the scales belong to the buyer and the seller has no way of checking on their accuracy. Cloth is also owned by the man, but he uses this to pay directly for goods and services rather than selling it for cash. Buyers may approach cloth owners and offer to buy so many arm-spans of cloth (the present price is approximately 50 cents per pound). A hunter will sell either fresh or dried meat in the evening by going around from house to house calling out that he has meat to sell. He will have cut the meat into pieces, roughly 1.5 kilograms each, and sell each piece for approximately 75 cents with no bargaining.

There are many more items that are the province of women to sell, but in the aggregate their value is much less than the things men sell. Women rarely, if ever, go around selling on their own, but rather they make up a tray or pan of things and price them for their children to sell. These items include, especially, palm nuts and peanuts, which children carry through the town. Women also do some selling from their homes. They may buy a 5-pound sack of salt or a tin of bouillon cubes from the Mandingo trader and resell smaller amounts of these. They place their wares on the ground in front of the house and leave a small child to watch over them. When a buyer comes along, who will usually be a child as well, the guardian calls the mother to conduct the sale. Soap and palm oil are also sold in this way.

Weaving

Of all the traditional types of work found in Gbarngasuakwelle, skilled work is in the most precarious position vis-à-vis cultural change. Virtually everything that was formerly made by hand can now be purchased in a machine-made version or substituted by a replacement that is of better quality and longer-lasting. As a result, contemporary Kpelle children may be opting not to learn and thus perpetuate these skills. Nevertheless, Gbarngasuakwelle appears to be unique among the many Kpelle towns I visited in valuing and keeping skilled work alive. There were people who claimed they preferred homespun to store-bought cloth and low wooden stools to chairs. These craft skills are complex; not everyone is invited to learn them, and we see here, most clearly, adults functioning as "teachers."

By far the largest category of skilled work is weaving. Weaving defines any construction activity that involves the intermeshing of plant fibers. The simplest form of weaving is thatching, where palm branches are simply overlapped one layer on top of another and then lashed to house rafter poles. Cloth weaving involves innumerable steps, many of which are quite difficult to master.

Cotton is planted by the male head of household on termite mounds that sprout throughout his rice farm. After it has been harvested, the cotton seeds are removed by rolling the balls under a heavy wooden or iron dowel. The balls, free of seeds, are then carded on a bow made of springy wood and strung with a leather thong. A handful of cotton is laid over the thong, which is then plucked. As the thong vibrates, dirt is shaken out and the fibers are loosened. When a household has accumulated a fairly large store of clean, unmatted cotton, the wife or wives spin it into yarn. Spinning is done by two or more women, mostly for companionship, as it is a one-person operation. The woman sits on the ground with her legs extended out in front of her. In her left hand she holds up a ball of cotton, and the fibers are spun onto a spindle which she manipulates with her right hand. The spindle is a tapered stick about 25 centimeters long with a removable clay whorl about 6 centimeters about the tip. The spinner sets the spindle in motion by rubbing the top of it between her palm and right thigh.

Some of the warp threads are dyed (*yee-tei*) an indigo blue, and when used with undyed threads, produce a striped pattern. Leaves of the *Gaay* tree are beaten in a mortar, then dried in the sun. They are put in a woven bag and submerged in water for a week. When they are taken out, most of the water is wrung out. Meanwhile, a funnel-shaped frame is constructed from vines and lined with banana leaves. Pieces of *Goa* tree are burned (they produce alkali, which acts as a mordant) and the ashes are placed in the funnel. The *Gaay* leaves are put in a pot under the funnel and water is poured over the ashes until the pot is full. The pot is covered tightly with banana leaves (they are softened by heating over the fire). This stands for a week. Pieces of the *Goa* tree are boiled in water for an hour (probably tannic acid, also a mordant) then the liquid is poured over the *Goa* ashes in the funnel and it drips into the pot with the dye. The dye is then stirred with a forked stick until large globules rise to the surface. It stands for 3 days before the washed and dried thread is put in for 4 hours. Then the thread is taken out and dried, dipped again, and so on, until it is the required shade.

When the head of the household has accumulated enough full bobbins of yarn, he either invites a weaver to weave it into cloth or, if he can, weaves it himself. One full bobbin of yarn yields a piece of cloth about 15 centimeters wide and one arm-span long. The arm-span is measured by holding an end of cloth in each hand and then extending both arms straight out at the sides. Eleven of these lengths are sewn together to make up a spread. Usually a man will not begin weaving until he has enough yarn to make at least five spreads or 55 full bobbins. If someone else does the weaving for the head of household, he has to be fed during this period of work and he gets to keep 2 out of every 10 spreads he weaves. To prepare the warp three sticks are pounded into the ground. One stick is usually 30–60 meters away from the other two. A man walks back and forth between these sticks holding the unwinding bobbin out to his side. He keeps track of the number of turns by grouping them by fours, when he has eight sets of four, he pushes these threads down and bunches them and begins a second group of eight sets of four. These two groups of 32 threads are then kept separate as they will be threaded through the heddles in two harnesses. The warped threads are then tied off in two groups and the whole thing is rolled into a ball.

The next step is to thread the heddles. These are pissava twine loops suspended between wooden bats. Each heddle receives one thread and there are 32 of them on each harness. Ends are then threaded between the reeds of the beater. The beater has a rounded wood top whose shape conforms to a man's palm and the reed is made of flexible strips of bamboo. Again, the ends are tied off in two groups as they come out of the beater and this whole outfit of warp ball, harnesses, and beater can be conveniently wrapped up and stored until the loom is constructed.

Perhaps the most remarkable physical skill possessed by men and women is the ability to vertically raise heavy and, by no means perfectly cylindrical, logs high in the air and repeatedly bring them down in the same spot. Women do this with the pestle in the mortar and men do it in building houses, kitchens, and looms. The main support posts are sharpened on one end by a machete, then they are grasped slightly below the center of gravity and raised to the full extension of a man's arms and brought down with a thud into the ground. This is done repeatedly with the same pole until it has sunk far enough into the ground to be stable. The weaver uses a length of a straight-growing reed as a yardstick and level to position the corner support poles. When these are in place, slimmer poles are lashed in place to complete the frame. Finally, the poles from which the harnesses hang and the back beam are added.

The strip of cloth that is woven is only 15 centimeters wide and, given the inevitably crooked loom, this width is probably near the maximum that can be made. The harnesses are draped over the horizontal supports and two wooden treadles raise and lower them to open the shed. There is no warp beam; instead, the warp threads are stretched out their full length and weighted with a heavy stone, which is moved forward as the weaving progresses. The loom is abandoned to rot after use, but the harnesses, beater, and shuttle are saved for reuse. Like other skilled workers, the weaver attracts a crowd of spectators, especially children.

Of the other woven items, the woman's woven bag most closely resembles cloth weaving in construction. This is *bii paa*. The thin, papery skin of the palm leaf is stripped off and left to dry. Then these are split into smaller strips about 0.5 centimeters wide and 1 meter long. The bottom of the bag is anchored to a porch-support pole and the bag is then woven in a circular fashion so that the weft strips form an upward moving spiral. There are two to four pairs of harnesses, depending on the ultimate size of the bag; as in the loom, the harnesses are raised and lowered to open a shed through which weft strips are passed. The weft strips are kept taut by passing them under the buttocks. Traps, mats, baskets, and other types of bags are woven by lifting the warp strips by hand. With each pass of the weft strip the weaver must raise alternate warp strips. Beating is done with the edge of the hand with the fingers extended.

Mats are the most frequently woven items. The warp strips are slivers of bamboo bark; the weft is palm leaf. The usual size is 1.3 meters × 2 meters. Slings and belts are braided, nets are crocheted, and hammocks are macraméd. For these latter two, twine must be made by twisting green stringy fibers from the pissava palm leaf between one's thigh and the palm of the hand. For nets, this continuous twine is woven onto a spiral frame made of the springy spine of the palm branch. The net is conical, with the apex at the bottom, and expands to a diameter of nearly 1 meter, when finished. A supporting ring of wood is left in the top, but the frame is removed. A hammock maker first prepares his twine, which is done in the same way as for a net, but it must be thicker. Then, using a memorized pattern, he constructs the hammock from a single continuous strand, using four types of knots to create the structure.

The woven cloth strips are sewn together and made into two types of men's garments. The first is a simple ankle-length robe with a square hole for the head to fit through. The second is a shorts and pullover combination. Women wrap a large piece of the cloth around themselves—usually from waist to ankles—the ubiquitous lappa. Blanket-size pieces are used as a night covering and are often used in brideprice payments or in settling other debts. Women use their bags to carry clean rice. Men use theirs to carry tools. Fanners are used in winnowing rice and also serve as drying trays for peppers. Other types of baskets have specific uses, such as the chicken basket. Palm thatch is loosely woven into a kind of universal carrier that is preferred for carrying clothing and unboiled rubber. Woven traps include fish traps and fence traps. Mats are used for sleeping and sitting and as a ground cloth on which rice, coffee beans, cocoa, and so on are spread to dry. Braided slings are used in the battle against rice birds. Almost every woman weaves nets and uses them for fishing. Hammocks are used for relaxing, by stringing them between two porch-support poles, and as stretchers for carrying sick or injured persons.

Other Crafts

We now turn to other types of skilled work. One characteristic of traditional wood carving is that it is highly utilitarian. Unlike other African societies, in which the carver occupies an important social position and decoration is lavished even on the most plebeian objects, carving in Gbarngasuakwelle is not highly esteemed. This does not mean that there is no decoration or aesthetics. Stools and combs, for example, are frequently incised with geometric designs. A short-bladed machete is used to hack the rough shape out of the wood. The choice of wood is very important. The *Bele* tree is preferred for doors, the *Basii* tree for mortars, *Nawo* for pestles, and so on. Once the shape is free, a short-handled adze finishes the roughing-out operation. For doors and mortars, little further effort is required. For more intricate pieces such as spoons and combs, the finishing work is done with a knife and the sanding with scaly leaves. Finally, the items are oiled. I found no evidence of *Pokoŋ*, or image carving. This work may be done in secret, or, which seems more likely, the term may refer to the sculpture of other neighboring tribes whose masks and figures are familiar to the Kpelle through their participation in the *Poro*.

Leatherwork has diffused from Saharan Africa and passed into Liberia from Guinea. Yɛlɛkɛ (whose name means skill), one of my principal informants, was the only leatherworker in the village, and he learned his trade from a Guinean. Using untanned skins is probably not new, but tanning, working, and dying the leather has been introduced. Untanned skins can be made into machete sheaths and hats. Snakeskins and leopard fur, in particular, are glued or sewn onto such ceremonial objects as fly whisks, the sacred headdress and spears used in warfare. Yɛlɛkɛ, because his legs are vestigial, must leave the hunting and skinning to his sons, and his friend tans the skins in two large clay pots which Yɛlɛkɛ made for this purpose. Before tanning he must scrape the hair, fat, and tissue away. Then he kneads the leather, like dough, to soften it. One of the most elaborate products is the tooled leather knife sheath. Starting with an iron knife, which, with the one-piece blade and handle measures 35 centimeters, he makes a wooden sheath. Then he takes strips of old cloth and, smearing them on both sides with a paste made from boiled cassava leaves, wraps them around the sheath and handle to build up a shape over which the leather is laid. Using the cloth strips, he creates a knob on top of the handle and another on the bottom of the sheath, Then he sews and glues the leather over the cloth and, finally, using a punch, tools a design in the surface. Less elaborate items include sandals and pouches. He also makes an all-leather bag that resembles a woman's purse with shoulder strap and front flap. These bags are carried by men, especially *Ƶò-na*, and are used to hold medicines, money, and other important items. A skilled leatherworker may make the *Koli-kolo*, which is a ceremonial "top hat" covered with "Moroccan" leather, cowry shells, leopard fur, seeds, cloth, and Colobus monkey fur. To make this hat, the leatherworker first must be initiated into the secret society that uses it and then must learn its iconography.

The potter makes unglazed, sundried pots, pipes, cups, and plates, but this skill is most severely threatened by modern substitutions and I was unable to study it.

The blacksmith continues to thrive, however; there are two at work in Gbarngasuakwelle. There are probably three reasons for this: First, the blacksmith does not receive cash, but instead his customers incur an obligation to work for him in a *kuu* on his farm. Second, most men prefer the traditionally shaped machete, which is shorter and has a hook on the tip of the blade, to the imported variety, which is longer, lighter, and has a straight blade. The blacksmith also makes tools that, as yet, have no machine-made counterpart (e.g., curved knives used in whittling and the long knife the leatherworker sheathes). Finally, the blacksmith has traditionally high status because his tools are essential to rice farming. In a *Menà* oath-taking ceremony, chicken blood was dribbled over the blacksmith's own tools. I asked why and the explanation involved a long inferential chain leading from the successful and, one might say, sacred rice crop back to the tools that help make the tools used in preparing the rice farm. The blacksmith is usually invited to join various secret societies and his knowledge of medicine is frequently extensive.

The blacksmith is the only skilled worker with a permanent workshop. This is an open-walled building with a sharply pitched thatched roof. Inside, is a forge that consists of two earthen mounds separated by a narrow trough in which a fire of woodchips is laid. An assistant works two leather bags which force air through bamboo tubes down and out a small opening at the base of the fire. A large and smaller rock serve as anvils and the blacksmith uses a variety of hammers, punches, and tongs in his work. A customer brings both the iron and the wood to be made into the requested tool—a blacksmith does only bespoke work. Formerly, iron, which is plentiful in the region, was smelted in local furnaces (Thomasson, 1987), but this practice has died out. Scrap iron is presently used. Only old men knew the secrets of iron smelting and one had to be initiated into these secrets, as in the *Poro*.

Building Things and Fixing Up the Town

In rice farming, children have specific duties. In certain kinds of town work, including crafts, they must be spectators unless specifically selected for training. In this section we look at a loose collection of work activities where children are expected to "pitch in," where skill is less important than energy and motivation.

House building is one such communal project. The traditional house was round with a cone-shaped roof and had no windows and a single door. There is only one such house still standing in the town and it is inhabited by a man who may well be the oldest resident (Plate 4.3). The house is built on a packed mud foundation to keep it above the floods the rainy season brings. A stake is pounded into the center of the foundation platform and with a piece of rope attached and another stake tied to the

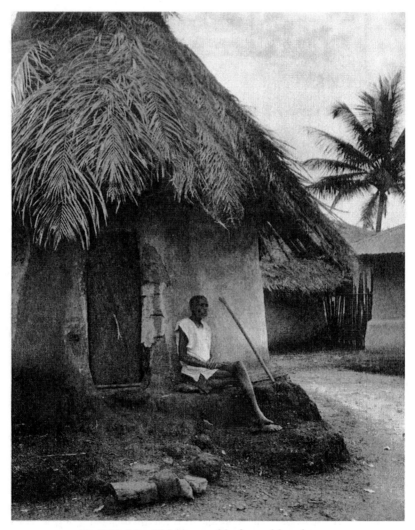

PLATE 4.3. Elder seated before oldest house.

free end of the rope, a circle is drawn in the dirt. Poles are sunk into the ground on the circumference in the manner described for loom building. These poles arc then lashed together with strips torn from a thick vine (Plate 4.4). Rafter poles are added and converge, teepee-fashion, at the top. Green palm branches are tied to these rafters and lap over each other. Branch ends are gathered together at the top and in a bundle bound tightly. A frame bench is fastened to the wall poles, which, once it is plastered,

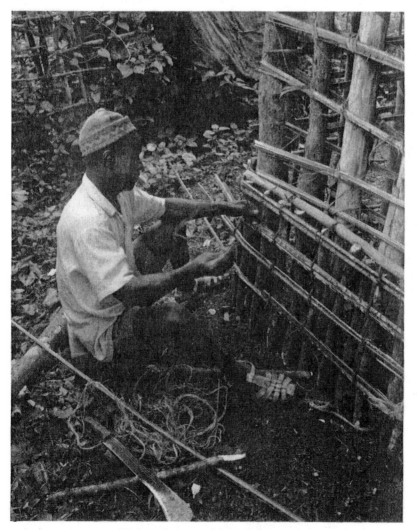

PLATE 4.4. Building a house.

serves as a bed. Clay-like soil is mixed with water and tramped underfoot to make a mortar which is flung onto the walls where it catches in the interstices of pole and vine. The mortar is put on both the inside and outside of the frame and when it dries, liquefied anthill mud is smeared on to provide a smooth, crack-free finish. Children assist with preparing palm thatch and plastering—a truly pleasurable type of work.

When completed, the wall is about 20 centimeters thick. These houses are small, about 5 meters in diameter at most, so a man typically owned more than one. Each of his wives and her children occupied a single house. The several households were not necessarily arranged in a compound; indeed, they may have been located at opposite ends of the town. Two other types of houses have been built in the last 40 years. The first is a modified cylinder with an arc of 30° sliced out to form a raised porch; otherwise this house is unchanged. A more radical departure is the rectangular house divided into two rooms and a porch. I was unable to ascertain just how people learned to build this house, which conceptually is far removed from the cylinder. For one thing, the roof peak has to be made quite differently.

The rafters in all of these houses serve as a storage area. Food, clothing, and so on are hung by rope or thongs in the center of the room, which makes them less accessible to rats. Cooking might be done in the center of the room or in a separate kitchen in the back.[3] A low fire is kept burning unattended under a drying rack or basket filled with venison or fish; on occasion, however, this fire may flare up, releasing large quantities of fat from the meat or fish which drips in the fire, and, in turn, sets off a conflagration. I witnessed one house burn under just such circumstances. There is no chimney; rather, the smoke filters through the thatch and undoubtedly acts as an effective insecticide. On farms the kitchens are built somewhat differently. Their main function is storage, so the roof portion is floored and the ratio of roof height to wall height is much higher than that of the in-town kitchen. The farm kitchen may also be unwalled. Kitchens for storing peanuts are rectangular with a gabled roof. Thatching is done by splitting the palm branch and tying halves lengthwise to horizontal roof members.

Domestic animals are ubiquitous in Gbarngasuakwelle, and the range of species includes chickens, ducks, guinea fowls, pigeons, sheep, goats, and dogs. They have free rein of the town so that they can scavenge for themselves in garbage dumps. These animals are rarely killed but, instead, serve as a storage for wealth and in payment of debts. Chicken, goats, and especially sheep are used in sacrifices and may be killed and eaten on other special occasions (e.g., the visit of "big men" such as the paramount chief) to show respect. Milk and eggs are not used by the owners. There is little work associated with animals except indirectly, which involves building fences to keep the animals out of gardens and "backyards." To the extent that animals are tended at all, they may be under the nominal care of children.

The principal activity that is identified as town cleanup is *naa fala*, or cutting grass. When a man says "this quarter is dirty," he is not referring to the rotting garbage, the cans and bottles, or the accumulated excrement of infants and domestic animals but, rather, to the sparse blades of grass that somehow manage to sprout in the otherwise unbroken mud flats. One of the principal duties of the quarter chief is to monitor this hirsute growth and cajole the householders in his quarter into getting rid of it. Women and children dig out this grass with short-handled hoes and pile it onto round-woven trays made specifically for this purpose to carry and dump beyond the town's perimeter. The seriousness with which this activity is treated was underscored when Namu (the chief masked "spirit" of the *Poro*) put in an appearance one morning and called all the initiated men and boys to clean a large, neglected area of the town as he looked on. A fair number of the large variety of snakes in Liberia are poisonous and by keeping the town free of grass, the danger they represent can be minimized. A person's first reaction on seeing a snake is to kill it. This practice must be a long-standing one because the snake population around Gbarngasuakwelle appears to be extinct or near extinct. On the other hand, the excrement from larger domestic animals, such as goats, sheep, and dogs represents a lethal danger to a populace who typically go shoeless. However, because the animals have only been recently introduced, the potential hazard is not yet appreciated.

MAKING MEDICINE

Medicine represents a paradoxical area of the society. It is open to change and innovation, and yet it is closed to inspection. With my small first-aid kit I was literally swamped with requests for medicants by people who had no reason to trust me and who had never used any kind of Western medicine before. Furthermore, as the following discussion shows, many traditional but foreign medicines and medical institutions have been introduced into the town and readily accepted. Medicine is closed in the sense that virtually all medicine is covered by *ifa mo*, which means "don't talk it," it is secret. To illustrate, I asked Yɛlɛkɛ, one of my most helpful sources, to give me the names of people conversant with trapping, weaving, and medicine making so that I could pursue my studies in these areas. He gave me the names of trappers and weavers but refused to name someone who knew medicine. I badgered him a little and he told me to see the chief. I proceeded to the chief who said he would look into it. Three weeks later Kerkula, a man I had never seen before, stopped at the house to introduce himself. A little later in the conversation he let out that someone had sent him a message that I wanted to learn about medicine making, He did not know who had sent the message and before answering any questions he told me what he would not talk about (which was quite a bit). Although he freely admitted to being a *Ẓò* (roughly, medicine man) who knew lots of medicine, if someone else had pointed this out it would have been a transgression against Kerkula, and one does not cross a *Ẓò*. There are sanctions against direct or indirect disclosures of medicine or anything associated with it.

To be sure, there are some nonsecret medicines, such as *loŋtuma*, which is a children's medicine, and *pala-sali*, which is for sores. These are widely known and applied and women, especially, seem to have a stock in trade of remedies for their children's illnesses. One of the most commonly used is a chalk-like paste for pain which is smeared on the skin (Plate 4.5). A few medicines are taught to children in the *Poro* and *Sande* bush schools; more important, children are supposed to learn respect for medicines and those who make them. The average individual does not, however, treat himself or even seek treatment until he is incapacitated by illness, a sore, an infection, and so on, and medicine does seem to be firmly in the hands of a few knowledgeable individuals. *Fenlee-la* is midwifery and although this is not secret to women, it is supposed to be closed to the scrutiny of men. Both divining and oath taking have secret or indecipherable elements but are, in fact, practiced publicly by specialists.

Sand cutting (divination) is done when someone is sick and the cause unapparent, when someone "acts funny," which could mean insanity or simple contrariness, or when something has been lost. The sandcutter runs his finger or a stick through loose sand spread out in a rough arc on the ground and interprets the patterns or tracks left in it. He makes a diagnosis, then the sick party or a person representing the sick party must go to someone who knows medicine for the cure. The term "sand cutting" has been retained to describe a variety of divining techniques some of which may have been recently introduced. One such procedure requires the sick person to lie down, then the diviner sprinkles medicine (no further expla-

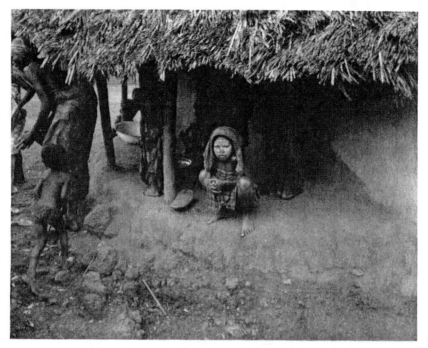

PLATE 4.5. Young girl with medicine on face.

nation given) on the person's forehead, says some garbled phrases, and commands the person to sleep. During sleep the dead ancestors appear to the person in a dream and tell him or her what is wrong. After 15 minutes, the diviner wakens the person and asks him or her to report on the conversation with the ancestors. I did not see this procedure executed, but from the description it appears as if the diviner is using hypnosis.

The ordeal (*jolo*) is also done publicly and probably derives much of its effectiveness from the presence of an audience. *Jolo* is used as a kind of lie detector test to determine whether the accused person or persons has committed a crime such as adultery, theft, destroying property, and so on. Like sandcutters and *Zò-na*, the *jolo* specialist enjoys a reputation that transcends village boundaries. There is one such specialist in Gbarngasuak-welle. In *yee-kan jolo*, the specialist smears a belt with medicine and wraps this around the bare waist of the accused, then says, "If this person is innocent let this belt remain as it is, if guilty, let it turn into an earthworm." Then the specialist cross-examines the person, touching on the issues in question. During this time, presumably, the belt has a chance to turn into an earthworm. I suspect that the perspiration brought on by nerves reacts with the "medicine," causing painful itching and burning, and a welt is raised where the belt rubbed against the skin, which, of course, resembles an earthworm. A second type of *jolo* was filmed in 1969 by James Gibbs in the nearby town of Fokwelle. This is *koli-gbolu* (hot iron) *jolo*. The specialist smears medicine on some part of his or a spectator's body, usually the leg or mouth. Then a red-hot machete is passed over this spot, which, in an innocent person, causes no burning. Then the same procedure is applied to the accused person or persons who have been watching the proceedings. I was told that a confession is usually forthcoming before the specialist has a chance to lay on the hot iron (several other types of ordeals practiced by the Kpelle are reported in Lancy, 1975a).

Kpo-loi is the name given to any place an individual habitually goes to make his medicine. Medicines are named for the purpose to which they will be put, that is, by the name of a sickness, such as *koi-puu* (diarrhea), the name of a situation, such as *jolo* or some other objective, such as *nyee-paa sali* which is for killing fish. Medicines are usually made from leaves, bark, berries, roots, and other wild flora and these are mixed, dried, beaten, fermented, and so on and may be applied internally or externally. The sick person is also told to avoid eating certain foods that might interfere with the medicine. An individual who has no claims to being a *Zò* may know several medicines. These are handed down from parent to favorite child when the parent is older or taught to a grateful patient. An individual who is sick or who has a sick child makes discreet inquiries as to who might know a medicine to cure the particular symptoms. The grapevine eventually carries the news to the person who knows the medicine. This person then has the option of ignoring the request or responding to the call and paying a visit to the ill person. The healer will ignore the call if he has some reason to dislike the sick person or does not know him. The healer is protected by his anonymity so that he cannot be identified by the sick person or his or her family unless he chooses to disclose himself. It should be pointed out that each symptom is treated as a separate sickness, or, in some cases, the most discomforting symptom, say, fever in the case of malaria, is treated and the others are ignored. If the diagnosis is straightforward or if a diviner has been consulted and the healer has stepped forward with the medicine, several courses are open to the patient. If the cure works, the patient is obliged to visit the healer and offer white Kola nuts, meaning a small gift to show respect and gratitude. If the medicine does not seem to be working, the sick person, if he or she can afford it, may consult a *Zò* or a member of a secret society whose pharmacopoeia is both more potent and more extensive. More on group secret medicine follows, but I would like to offer a short list of medicine names so that the reader will get some idea of the range of situations in which medicines are applied.

1. *Foloŋ-sali*, medicine to cure an illness brought on by violating a taboo against having sexual intercourse during the day; usual symptoms are pain or swelling of the genitalia.
2. *Bare-sali*, a class of medicines that aid in luring animals into traps.
3. *Ma-tee sali*, medicine to remove a sickness in children. The child has trouble walking and running. In a child the cause is violation of the taboo against sexual intercourse prior to puberty. In an infant it signals a violation of the taboo against the mother having intercourse before her baby can walk.
4. *Moleŋkpe sali*, medicine to drive away evil spirits.
5. *Kpamo-sali*, medicine to remove *kpamo*. Sympathetic magic where an individual takes an enemy's lock of hair, piece of clothing, fingernails, and so on, and burns them or buries them. The former causes the enemy to suffer fever, the latter to have trouble breathing. *Kpamo-sali* is made only after a diviner has ascertained the true cause of the illness.
6. *Meni nɛɛ sali*, a class of medicines for luck, in gambling, in love, with a rice crop, and so forth.
7. *Koi-gbala*, a laxative.
8. *ŋee-sali*, a local anesthetic used when one has a toothache.

In studying group secret medicine, the doctrine of *ifa mo* applies in force. I had to attack in a roundabout way and most of my information came in a series of general statements given as answers to a hypothetical question, "What would happen if the chief got very sick?" Answers to this question gave me a tantalizing glimpse of the natural, social, political, and psychological forces that are both stimulated and controlled by Kpelle medicine. In the first place, the chief, because of his role as judge, can be expected to make a few enemies. Chief Wollokollie on another occasion, gave this as a principal reason why he did not like being town chief. These enemies may "curse one's name," may make *kpamo* against one, or poison one's food. Second, as chief, he would be open to the sin of pride. This is, of course, my own interpretation, but it fits well with what I was told, which was that a man cannot push his destiny; he should not try to outdo his ancestors, his peers, or the devils, (i.e., Namu and others), at least not flagrantly. If he does, evil spirits will be set to work to bring about his destruction. Third, the chief, unlike the average man, must expose himself. The average villager, from my perspective, is taciturn and suspicious and hides away in the town, the quarter, and his house—he avoids contacts with those he does not know intimately. The chief, by virtue of his office, cannot afford this luxury and must get involved with people who are relative strangers to him, even if they have lived their whole lives in Gbarngasuakwelle. All these strangers are a possible source of danger.

The best analogy I can think of to illustrate this attitude is that of the doctor making rounds in the hospital. He must expose himself to any number of contagious diseases. The Kpelle do not have a germ theory of disease, but they do believe that someone with evil ways or evil thoughts can do subtle harm, there are bad men and these people are best avoided. With strangers one never knows, but Wollokollie must face them all. My informants agreed that Wollokollie would be an unlikely violator of sexual taboos or *ifa mo* in connection with the *Poro* or other secret societies of which he was a member. Any of these offenses could bring on sickness, but given Wollokollie's character, which must be taken into account in any diagnosis, these possibilities could be safely ruled out. So much for the forces of evil; clearly, any outspoken enemies of the chief would be primary targets of suspicion, but the investigation would probably be long and complex.

The forces of good are equally formidable, as my informants avowed that the loss of Wollokollie would be a blow to the town. He could expect constant attention from his wives and children and offers of help from everyone in his quarter. As a member of at least three secret societies besides the *Poro*, the *Nia* (witch-hunting), *Gborbiliŋ* (millipede), and *Kali-sali* (snake) societies, he could count on a vast range of medical expertise. One of the prime functions of these societies is the protection of their own members and the untimely death of Wollokollie would diminish their reputation. The *Ƶò-na* would also be out to enhance their reputations as powerful healers, and would welcome an opportunity to demonstrate their knowledge on such an important figure as the chief. Finally, if he were to die and his enemy were known, the *Poro* leaders might call *Loi-meni saa*, and the culprit might ultimately be dispatched by the *Goi-manaŋ* (banana sap society).

Secret societies are powerful and pervasive in Gbarngasuakwelle, but, unfortunately, due to the doctrine of *ifa mo*, it was extremely difficult to elicit information about them. However, there are a number of cultural routines implicated in learning Kpelle medicine, as we learn from Bellman's (1975, 1983) extensive work on sorcery—including his own initiation into one of the secret societies.

CONCLUSION

We can look on the work taxonomy as a kind of college course catalog. Rice farming is like general education—required of everyone—although there is considerable differentiation of role as a function of age and gender. Hunting, trapping, fishing, and gathering function as electives; no one enforces children's acquisition of these skills. Talking matter reflects something akin to a generic set of skills—composition or speech—that are acquired along the way. Weaving and other skilled work represent advanced, specialized courses—not open to all—with many prerequisites. As will become clear in the chapters that follow, the average Kpelle masters only a small fraction of this curriculum.

In this chapter we have considered the end points of the enculturation process—adults, through their many skills, constructing a complex and viable community. To follow children along the various pathways to those end points, in the next chapter we begin at or near the beginning by observing infants and toddlers at play. In Chapters 6 and 7 we continue to examine the enculturative effects of various playforms—with progressively older children. In Chapter 8 we look at the origins of "real work" showing how early in the child's development they are given responsible chores. Then, in Chapter 9 we look at older children as they learn the attributes of adulthood through increasingly formal means.

Parents, Children, and Make-Believe

. . . the child grows up in a crowded and intricate organizational
world whose features he has to learn.

—OTTENBERG (1989, p. xxi)

PORTRAITS OF KPELLE LIFE

Daylight was breaking as the women and children gathered at the corner
near the road. By 7:00 A.M., they had set out down the road with babies on
their backs and pots, pans, and tools on their heads. After walking some 3.5
kilometers they cut off into the bush and soon came to a clearing. They
walked to an area where several large trees had been cut down. There they
deposited their burdens and, taking up their hoes, proceeded to work in a
line, loosening the soil with quick jabs at the ground. They worked fast but
paused frequently to straighten up, catch their breaths, and refasten their
lappa skirts, which were slipping open. The *kuu* was working on Nangbo's
farm and she was in charge of baby minding and cooking. The dead trees
formed a convenient kind of playpen and most of the 14 children played
there and on the logs. She frequently scolded them for climbing on the slip-
pery trunks and running out of the area, She sent two 7-year-old girls to
gather wood and water and she cleared an area for the fire. Her husband,
Kollie, had arrived and, with two of the 17 women, he cut down weeds with
a machete and gathered them in piles so the women hoeing would have a
clear field. One of the older women soon stopped and, taking a rice fanner,
filled it with the seed rice that Nangbo had given her and began broadcast-
ing handfuls of it onto the prepared ground. There were five infants, all but
two of whom spent the entire day on their mothers' back. These two were
taken care of by older sisters, ages 7 to 8, who brought them to the mother
periodically for feeding. The infants, whether on their mothers' or older sisters' back, slept most of the time (Plate 5.1).

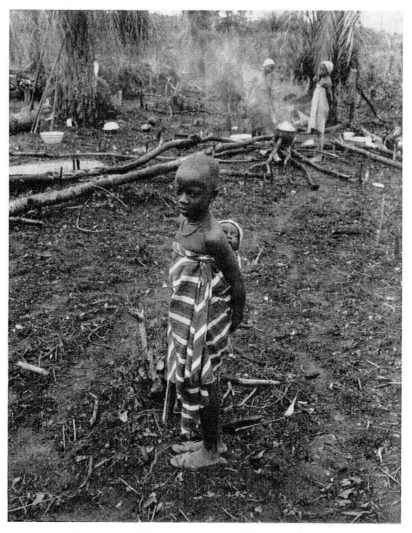

PLATE 5.1. Girl carrying infant on her back.

Nangbo had gotten a fire started and was cooking rice in two large cast-iron pots; as she stirred the rice she kept an eye on the children around her who were, at this time, getting a little restless. Lorpu, Kollie's brother-in-law, had come and he was cutting stakes for a fence that would surround the farm. The working women chattered and joked to each other and occasionally one would break into a song. The three teenage unmarried women worked together and there were other clusters of women.

Two boys, ages 8 and 9, played a spirited game of tag in an adjacent field that had been planted during the past week. They were supposed to be chasing birds from the rice seed but had to be reminded of this by their mother, who was busy weaving a sling in the partially completed kitchen. Their game served the same purpose, however, as they careened, yelling from one end of the farm to the other, and thus they were effective deterrents to the birds. At 11:00 A.M., the rice was cooked and everyone stopped working. The women washed off their faces and hands from the water bucket and took their first drink of the morning, then sat on the logs and passed over their bowls to be filled. Now they were very quiet, but the children were activated by this break in the routine and became much more lively. Mothers ate as babies nursed and toddlers backed themselves between their mothers' knees. The 7-year-olds took this opportunity for a little game of tag themselves. By 11:30, they all began to work again.

Tomorrow this scene will be repeated on another of the *kuu* members' farms, and so on until all the farms have been planted.

This vignette should provoke the same sort of reaction as Bruegel's depictions of animated scenes from Flemish village life. It is, in fact, rather idyllic. People's actions intermesh in a mutually supportive fashion. Here women do not have to choose between work or child care. There is no lengthy negotiation about what each person will do that day, there is no "back talk," no cajoling, no promise of reward for "being good." The "script" that guides the behavior of Kpelle of all ages is, with some notable exceptions (Bellman, 1983), a remarkably open book.

Here is a similar scene in town: It is late in the afternoon and three women and a girl of 7 are seated on the ground in front of the house. The head of the household is seated on the edge of a bench, which adjoins the house. Two of his small children, a boy and a girl, ages 2 and 3, are playing under, around, and on top of the bench. Of the women, two are wives of the man and a third, who lives nearby, is a sister of one of the wives. The women gossip as they shell and partially consume the peanuts. Fifty feet away, a third wife sits by the kitchen, her head cradled in her hands, she is ill, probably with malaria. The man watches and periodically he and his 10-year-old son, who has been sitting next to him, take pans full of shells to the edge of the town and dump them. The children play with a small pan that has a hole in the bottom. The little girl puts empty shells in the pan, then dumps them out, she does this repeatedly. Tiring of this, she bangs the pan on the little boy's head; he takes it from her and wears it as a hat. The little girl starts to scream and one of the women tells him to give it back, which he does. One of the wives scoops shelled nuts into a fanner and begins bouncing it up and down as shell fragments fly out on the ground. This noise stimulates the little girl with the pan to mimic the bouncing action with the shells in her pan, which she does perfectly even though her back has been turned to the adults the whole time. In the kitchen a baby wakes up and starts to cry. The 7-year-old girl goes to fetch it and attaches it to her back with a length of cloth. The infant's mother takes the baby from its older sister's back and begins to nurse it. Another daughter joins the group; she is about 10. She brings her own pan and gets it filled with unshelled nuts but does not sit down with the group. Instead, she goes and sits down beside her mother, the sick woman, and begins shelling; the two exchange no conversation. A short while later it starts to rain and everyone prepares to retire indoors. The neighbor-woman holds out her hands, the headwife fills them with shelled nuts, and she leaves. The women carry their pans and stools inside and the man and his son make one last trip to dump the shells.

Again we see the complex, interlocking web as an extended family undertakes the task of shelling and cleaning peanuts. Child care and socialization are integrated fully into these other routines. With the exception of one directive—telling the boy to return the pan—there is little evidence of the sort of active parenting found in our own society. Indeed, as we see in a later section, even very young children, are free from the constant scrutiny of their parents. They are most often to be found "playing on the mother-ground." That is, they play in open areas between houses and are subject to the casual scrutiny of a number of adults, not limited to their biological parents, who happen to be within range.

"Parenting," "child rearing," and "educating" are all but invisible in Kpelle society; hence, it was difficult to elicit a widely shared version of how these things were to be done. However, the notion of "good child versus bad child" provided an appropriate starting point.

KPELLE EXPECTATIONS FOR CHILDREN

I conducted a group interview with three men and three women ages 30 to 40, all of whom had several children. Excerpts from that interview follow[1]:

QUESTION: What does a good child do?
FIRST MAN: A child who has good ways will imitate his father. If his father is a trapper, he will learn to make a trap. If his father is a palm wine maker, he will learn how to make palm wine.

SECOND MAN: As the way I play *Fanga* [a type of drum] my children will learn it. If I'm cutting brush, I give him the machete for him to know how to cut brush. If work becomes hard, I'll show him how to make it easier.

FIRST WOMAN: The work I do she will do some of it. She will plant rice, beat rice, and draw water.

[Spontaneously, the men interpreted the question as referring to their sons whereas the women spoke only of their daughters.]

THIRD MAN: We will teach our children our work. We will tell them, "If one learns this type of work, one's life will be longer." If a child listens to you and you explain things to him, he will give you no cause for anger. If a child doesn't obey you or if you don't advise him, he will cause you shame in front of your friends. A good child makes people praise his father's name.

FIRST MAN: If you have a child who is good, people will come to you and say, "This child gives respect to old people, he doesn't abuse anyone, he's a nice boy." A good father will have a good child.

FIRST WOMAN: What makes a child good? If you ask her to bring water, she brings water. If you ask her to cook she cooks, if you tell her to mind the baby, she does it. When you ask her to plant rice she doesn't complain.

[A good child, then, is one who does family work willingly, is loyal and obedient to his father/mother, and shows respect toward older people.]

QUESTION: What does a bad child do?

FIRST MAN: "A bad child shows his mother's buttocks" [proverb meaning that a bad child is born from his mother's anus rather her vagina].

THIRD MAN: If a child is very bad, it is hard for his father to eat. You can't go among your friends with a bad child because you will be ashamed. Such a person's ways follow him forever.

SECOND MAN: If a child is a thief you won't acknowledge him as your son. If he's good many people will claim him as their son.

FIRST MAN: It is the devil [said in English] that put these ideas in his head, for such a person, you will go to a sandcutter [diviner] to find out what makes this boy so bad. The sandcutter will tell you what to do about the child.

THIRD MAN: You have a woman [i.e., your wife], she will have intercourse with another man, a bad man. The child will copy the bad man.

They say you're the father and you wonder why your child is bad. You don't know about the woman and the bad man [apparently a belief that goodness or badness may be inherited].

SECOND WOMAN: A girl who is trained will take her mother's steps, if her mother can make fishnet or spin thread, she will learn it from her mother. She won't leave the house while she is cooking to go and play.

THIRD MAN: If someone gives you an old house you take care of it and make it new again. Sometimes they bring a bad child to you to raise it and you can sometimes make it good.

[Children, then, are influenced, primarily by the same-sex parent; they are expected to follow their "steps." Boys are more likely to go bad than girls, probably because they have more freedom and fewer responsibilities than girls. Badness may be reversible when a good man takes on a bad child to raise. The first man in this interview worked as a jitney driver and this necessitated his being away from home for days at a time. His 9-year-old son was becoming "bad" and he came to me to help him compose a letter to his former employer asking this man to take and raise the boy.]

QUESTION: What do you do if a child refuses to work?

SECOND MAN: [Referring to young men] Some spend all day in town, just passing up and down. They don't want to do farmwork. If a child doesn't work on the farm, you beat him. If he still won't go, you bring no food for him into the town. If he sleeps hungry, he'll go on the farm the next day.

THIRD MAN: If a child doesn't want to go on the farm I'll send him to school. If the child can't do anything, I can't accept.

SECOND MAN: If I show him all the different kinds of work we do and he doesn't want to work, I'll send him to school and if he doesn't want to learn I'll let him go wherever he wants.

A brief anecdote is in order to support and underscore the themes addressed in the interviews. Shortly after I arrived in Gbarngasuakwelle, a boy of 16 presented himself to me as a houseboy. I was warned that he was a bad boy and that I should have nothing to do with him. Nevertheless, he was rather droll and seemed earnest so I hired him. In the course of time, he gave me cause to regret my decision. He stole from me, he argued with me when I asked him to do some work, and people were constantly coming to complain that he had abused them and called them foul names. In other words, he demonstrated the three principal traits of the bad boy as brought out in the interview. So pervasive is this concern for children who lack respect for elders and traditions that an English word "frisky" has come in to widespread parlance throughout Liberia to describe this "type." According to Erchak (1977), adults rationalize clitoridectomy (a prominent feature of *Sande* initiation) for a girl by saying it reduces her friskiness, thus making her "more easily controlled by her husband . . ." (p. 127).

I had occasion to meet other "bad" boys and they seemed all to have deceased, absent, or "bad" fathers. One boy of 8 was nothing less than a pesky nuisance and greatly hampered my work. When I complained about him to other people I was told, "What do you expect, his father's a bad man who always abuses and runs after women." Bad children are the exception rather than the rule. So parents influence children by example and by setting limits on their behavior, but not through direct *teaching*.

Why the Kpelle Do Not See Themselves as Their Children's Teachers

Although all societies have routines for preparing children to become adults, there are broad differences in the "mix" between such Western, industrialized societies as our own and more traditional agrarian, pastoral, and foraging societies. The need to prepare children to succeeed in an increasingly demanding and lengthening system of formal education places a greater burden on parents and fuels a veritable culture routine industry. Rogoff (1990) reviews at length cases of middle-class parents who provide all sorts of guidance, scaffolding (cf. Wood, Bruner, & Ross, 1976), and instructional conversations while noting that, in non-Western cultures, there is much less evidence of parents doing these things. Then she proceeds to chastise middle-class parents for stressing independence and individuality, for encouraging children "to rely not on people for comfort but on pacifiers, blankets and other 'lovies'" (p. 208). She does not see that the resolution of this contradiction lies in acknowledging that middle-class parents expect much more of their children[2] than do lower-class parents or parents in non-Western societies (see also Tudge, Putnam, & Sidden, 1993). These heightened expectations mean that these children's lives will be extra stressful and they will need much more comforting than children whose parents demand far less of them. Here is a recent bromide under the headline "Teach Preschoolers More, Studies Say":

... By the time he enters kindergarten at age 5, it may be too late to catch up. You can spot a dropout as early as kindergarten. ... This is not a time when you can just let a child be babysat until they're more alive and more interesting. ... There's a real job for parents to do, and it's not just hanging around to make sure their child doesn't eat poison. (Gannett News Service, 1992, p. A14)

Further, the emphasis on independence as opposed to cooperation and interdependence (which Rogoff advocates) sends the following message to the child: "We expect you to rise above other children, to strive to do *your* best rather than to do only what others around you are doing."

As noted throughout this volume, Kpelle adults do *not* see themselves as their children teachers, and for good reason. The mother may be too busy to spend much time with her children. In many societies, including the Kpelle, not only do women have prime responsibility for child rearing and maintenance of the household, they are the primary food producers as well. Given high infant mortality rates, parents may be unwilling to make a large investment in a child who might die. Responsibility for child rearing is diffuse; parents are only two among many caretakers—indeed, the father is not usually among the more prominent caretakers—who include siblings, extended family members, and neighbors.

There seems to be little need to "accelerate" development because there is far less information to acquire; in particular, parents do not have to ensure that their children will become literate.[3] The tasks to be learned are relatively simple and do not require elaborate "schooling." Nothing in the Kpelle child's environment is as complicated as a bicycle, let alone an erector set.[4] To the extent that we understand folk theories of child development, these theories are at variance with our own. Although we believe in adjusting situations to fit the child—*Tomee Tipee* cups[5]—Kpelle adults, as those in most other societies, believe children must adapt to situations or avoid situations they are not mature enough to handle. Also, although we believe in actively creating "age-appropriate" learning environments for children—think of those minigyms that fit on the rails of a baby's crib—the Kpelle (see also quote from Heath in Chapter 2) see observation and imitation of adults as the most appropriate curriculum for children. To return to a notion introduced earlier, we tend to be "optimizers" vis-à-vis the preparation of children for adulthood, whereas most of the rest of world tend to be "satisficers" (cf. Simon, 1956).

Adult–Child Interaction and Teaching
"Proper" Speech and Manners

As noted in Chapter 2, the exception to the rule that parents in non-Western societies do not self-identify as teachers is the teaching of manners. First, one must consider the age of the child. The Kpelle distinguish between different stages (e.g., *siye-long* = around 6 months, not walking yet; *sia-long* = toddler; *surong long* = little boy) and expectations for child and caretaker behavior vary systematically with age. Wrapped in a cloth sash, infants are, marsupial-like, attached to their mother for the first 6 months and are fed on demand.[6] Not until children can walk are they granted limited autonomy from the mother's person (Plate 5.2). Obviously adaptive for mother and infant, this approach keeps the mother's hands free for working and spares her infant the inevitable hazards that crawling on the ground would expose it to. Although the mother is the sole caretaker of the newborn, as the child gets older he or she will be handled, and, occasionally, played with, by its mother, father, siblings, and other extended family members.[7] Contrary to the prevailing view of language socialization in the West, one does not see any sort of "conversation" with the infant (see also Ochs & Schieffelin, 1984, on the situation in Samoa and New Guinea). Observational studies (Field et al., 1981) have demonstrated that whereas mothers in the United States often hold their infants in the *en face* position—to facilitate communication— this is rarely done by mothers elsewhere. Similarly, LeVine and LeVine (1981), from their work in East Africa, note:

> Our Gusii data show that after their infants are 3 months old the amount of eye contact permitted declines rapidly . . . infants . . . attempt to engage their mother in reciprocal play . . . mothers tend to ignore these efforts . . . For a mother to engage a small child, let alone an infant, "in conversation" would . . . seem eccentric behavior . . . since . . . a child is not a valid human being until he reaches the age of "sense" . . . six or seven years old. (pp. 43–44)

The situation does not change as children get older. Adults direct very little speech at children[8] except to correct their behavior, and then with only a brief reprimand. Nor are adults particularly prone to correct children's speech (Erchak, 1977). Further, although the Kpelle are concerned when children fail to show respect, there are no widely recognized routines to "instruct" children in proper etiquette. This is one area in which the Kpelle stand in sharp contrast to a number of other societies in

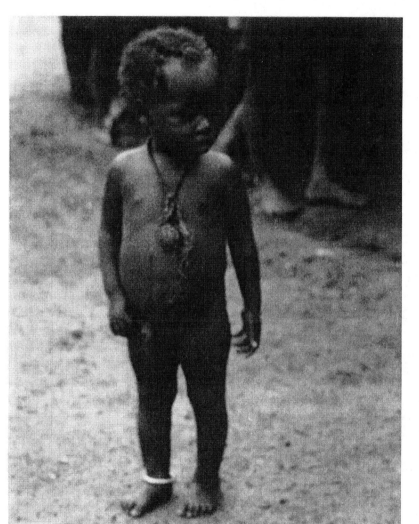

PLATE 5.2. Baby with amulet.

the ethnographic literature, which begin to train children in the intricacies of the social system from an early age.

"Arunta children learn the content of kinship terms as they interact daily with specific people. They are informed repeatedly by adults who individuals are and how they should act toward them" (Williams, 1972/1983, p. 202). In Samoa, "Very small children are encouraged to produce certain speech acts that they will be expected to produce later as younger (i.e., low ranking) members of the household. . . . [They] will be explicitly instructed to notice others and to provide information to others" (Ochs & Schieffelin, 1984, pp. 296–297). "The first and most important lessons which the [Navajo] child learns about human relationships are the approved ways of dealing with various classes of relatives" (Leighton & Kluckhon, 1948, p. 44). When they transgress, they "are told the big gray *Yeibichai* will carry them off and eat them" (Leighton & Kluchhon, 1948, p. 51). Kwara'ae "lecture" children using rhetoric normally reserved for rituals and meetings. These lectures invariably deal with rules for appropriate social behavior, especially the need to respect those of higher rank, including one's older siblings (Watson-Gegeo & Gegeo, 1986, 1989).

One of the most interesting cases of parent as teacher in the literature was documented by Bambi Schieffelin (1979, 1986) in her research among the Kaluli in the highlands of New Guinea. Kaluli mothers take an active part in teaching even infants proper speech forms to use with different audiences. They hold their young on their laps and, like a ventriloquist's dummy, make them "speak" to others passing by. Then, once the child has begun to speak, the mother utters a particular phase and instructs the child to repeat after her. The goal seems to be to teach children to use socially correct speech as rapidly as possible.

This catalog illustrates that although parents rarely engage in explicit teaching with their young children, when they do, the object of instruction seems, inevitably, to be the acquisition of kinship and politeness conventions (Firth, 1970). In fact, this appears also to be true in the West,[9] at least among poor and working-class families whose rare "lessons deal . . . with good behavior toward other people" (Tudge et al., 1993, p. 81).

Paying Attention

In the absence of direct instruction, how are children expected to learn proper behavior and skills? They learn through observation and imitation. Note in the epigram that opened the chapter, the phrase is "has to learn" rather than "will be taught." In our own society we put a premium on independence, assertiveness, innovation, and competition in our children. Parents often allow themselves to be duped or beaten by their young to encourage this sort of initiative and ambition.

My colleague David Bergin *proudly* relates that, as he was seated in a wooden chair, his 5-year-old son, Sam, was hanging off the back of it. He said, "Sam, stop doing that, you might pull the back off." Sam walked around to face his father and, with hands on hips, rejoined, "Well, I guess we'll just have a stool, then."

Rogoff (1990), by contrast, observes that: "in a Mayan community ... children are taught to avoid challenging an adult with a display of greater knowledge by telling them something" (p. 60).

We do not want our children "underfoot"; we want them to create and master their own universe. Our child-rearing procedures are adapted to the demands posed by an extremely complex and information-rich culture—a culture in which one can experience the failure of dropping out as early as 10. Much of what one needs to know in order to thrive in our society is, in effect, hidden in print material and specialized language. A part of Kpelle culture is also hidden; consequently, the society utilizes special procedures to enable individuals to gain access to it. However, the amount that is hidden compared to that which is open is relatively small and, furthermore, the average Kpelle—especially the average Kpelle woman— can function quite successfully in the society while having mastered only a fraction of this hidden culture (Bellman, 1983).

The Kpelle and other preindustrial cultures accomplish the education of their young through a much more natural and casual process. I have already suggested that Kpelle culture is public, accessible to all. Coupled with this fact we have what appears to be a universal tendency for the young to observe and imitate their elders, and so the job gets done (Katz, 1981). Meyer Fortes's (1970) classic study of enculturation among the Tallensi (Ghana) is replete with these sorts of observations: "Whatever I do [my son] also sits and listens. Will he not get to know it thus?" (p. 22); "... a capmaker told me how he learned his craft, as a youth ... by carefully watching [a capmaker] at work. When he was young, he explained, he had 'very good eyes'" (p. 23).

In Gbarngasuakwelle, the town chief holds "court" in one of the larger open areas of the town, and this truly resembles a kind of open-air Greek drama. The chief is seated on the porch of a house *above* everyone else. One by one those who testify parade across the "stage" in front of the chief. To either side of the open area, elders—the chorus—are seated on the verandah of adjacent houses. Every case I recorded was watched by a few children, usually seated on logs at the periphery of the stage. That even young children should find this worth watching amazed me, especially as most of the discourse could be described as "deep Kpelle" (cf. Bellman, 1983) and thus all but unintelligible to the young. Cross-cultural studies (Whiting & Edwards, 1988) have documented the enormous amount of waking hours young children spend in just watching. Could it be that our own youngsters' predilection for hours-long television gazing has ancient and adaptive origins?

Observing one's "betters" has been widely documented in the literature. Among primates, submissive or low-ranking animals spend far more time gazing at dominant individuals than the reverse. This phenomenon has been replicated with human children and even extended to the classroom—children who are successful, who usually have the right answers, are likely to attract the rapt attention of their peers, whereas academically weaker children tend to be ignored.

Rivalry between siblings seems also to be far rarer than in our society. Older siblings are specifically charged with the care of younger brothers and sisters and it seems clear that the younger ones invest what we might identify as filial affection in their big brothers and sisters. The apron strings that bind the youngster emotionally to its caretaker are as likely, in most societies, to be big sisters as mothers (Weisner & Gallimore, 1977). Further, there appears to be a general tendency for the younger generation to "idolize" the next older generation, especially when each older age cohort is afforded new privileges and responsibilities by the society (see especially Read, 1960). Zukow (1989) concludes her review of sibling caretaking: "In broad terms, younger siblings notice what their older siblings do, repeat it, and, in more goal-directed settings, follow their guidance" (p. 85).

ON THE MOTHER-GROUND

The most striking evidence that children are attending to and learning from others around comes from noting their make-believe play. In Kpelle this is *Neé-pele*, which not only refers specifically to make-believe but is also used, generally, to characterize the play of very young children. *Neé-pele* involves the conscious dramatization of some real-life and usually adult activity by children ages 4 to 11. A little boy carrying a bell chases after two little girls as they run round and round a kitchen. What are they doing? According to an informant, he is the dog and the girls are antelope. Men use small dogs, with bells tied around their necks, in hunting antelope. The children have never actually seen their fathers hunting in this manner, but they must have heard about it and are now reenacting the hunt. A group of four girls (two 6-year-olds, two 4-year-olds) are playing at pounding rice. They have built up conical piles of dirt (mortar) with a depression in the center. With slender sticks (pestle) about 1 meter long they "pound" into the depression in their dirt pile (Plate 5.3). This becomes a kind of dance as they lift their "pestles" in unison and make up a song about what they are doing. One girl scoops up sand in a dish and pretends to eat it. She brings the sand in her hand to her chin (mouth) and makes chewing movements with her mouth. Later they scatter around the square and hunt for "snails." (There are no snails in town.) They pick up rocks (snails), which they put in cans (pans) They balance the cans on their heads and walk around, trying alternately to balance the cans and then unbalance them so the rocks fall out. Then the two 6-year-olds take the 4-year-olds on their backs and play "mother." Continuously they weave dance steps and songs into their play. One song is "Mr. David, take my picture," and while singing it they dance [jump] around in a circle.

The children have been playing "on the mother-ground" (*panaŋ lè-ma*) (Plate 5.4). The phrase designates areas of the town where children habitually gather to play. This particular mother-ground is the area in front of the chief's house also used for the court. There are two other such areas in the town also in large open squares. These children were playing during the day, but this is somewhat unusual. Typically, play on the mother-ground is limited to the evening and moonlit nights, when children

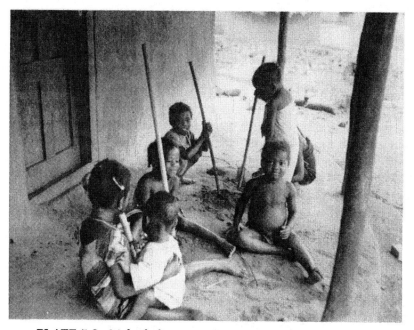

PLATE 5.3. Make-believe grinding with mortar and pestle.

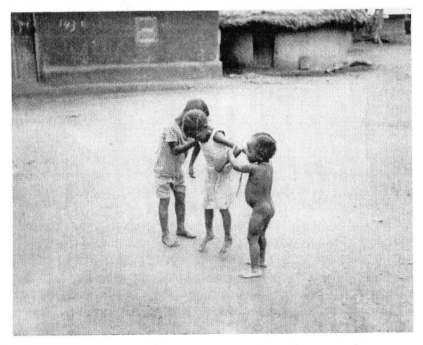

PLATE 5.4. Children playing on the mother-ground.

from the quarter gather for *Neé-pele*, dancing, and other play. These children were not on the farm this particular day because their mother was sick and stayed in the village.

The term "mother-ground" connotes an area where children can be "mothered" or watched over. As LeVine (1973) observed, it is a pan-African phenomenon that "children soon learn that any grownup can rebuke them and has authority over them" (p. 35).[10] Evidence of the existence in village-based societies of a mother-ground is widespread.[11] Among the Chaga, there is "a children's play area, often at the edge of or near the village commons" (Raum, 1940, p. 95). Williams (1969) observes of the Dusun: "while the adults present . . . tend to take little notice . . . of the children of these play groups . . . [they] tend to cluster in the areas near houses where an adult is present" (p. 75).

Situating play areas in close proximity to adults serves two ends. It affords older individuals the opportunity to oversee the children and also gives children a *source* of scenes to incorporate into their play. Imitation must be preceded by observation. Here is a representative sample of make-believe from Gbarngasuakwelle:

• Children on the farm make their own *kuu.* Boys sing and swing their sticks (machetes) at the weeds. Girls cook dirt (rice) in snail shells (pots) over sticks the boys have fetched for the "fire."

• A girl makes thread from pissava palm fibers (actually strips the fiber into threads rather than twisting it), which she winds onto a "bobbin." This she gives to a boy who has made a "loom" from bamboo sticks. He lays two sticks on the ground, parallel to each other to represent heddles, and moves his feet up and down as if to raise and lower them. Leaves or paper represent the woven cloth and this is divided up among the "children" for their "clothes."

• A few men from Gbarngasuakwelle have, at one time or another, gone down to the coast to work for a few months for wages on the Firestone rubber plantation. I observed a 7-year-old boy with his younger brothers and sisters reenacting the homecoming scene of a worker returned from Firestone. He had made a carrier basket of palm thatch and proceeded to distribute to his "wife and children": dirt (salt), leaves (clothes), sticks (shoes), rope (belt), gourds (pots), and cowry shells (money).

• Several boys ages 8 to 10 practice climbing palm trees, to "cut palm nuts." They play on a coconut tree which has a convenient curve in it not found in the oil palm tree, making it easier to climb the first few feet. Their *Baliŋ* is a strip of bamboo, which they loop around the trunk and hold at their sides (Plate 5.5).

PELE-SEŊ

A natural outgrowth of make-believe is the construction of "props." Sometimes, the props themselves, toys or *Pele-seŋ* (literally, play things), become the focus of attention. Machetes, hoes, hammers, and their make-believe counterparts are toys to young children in that, when they first begin to use the tools, they do so spontaneously, in the course of playing. A piece of cloth rolled into a bundle serves as a baby doll. A stick becomes a shotgun. Leaves and twigs are woven into mechanical puzzles, which stymie even the "smart" white man. Older children and men capture small animals, birds, and large insects; tie strings on them; and give them to small children to play with. A bird or large beetle is tied by its legs, leaving its wings free to move, and it flies, tethered, around and around the child's head. Small, furry rodents are fed, petted, cuddled, then traded or sold by their owners to another curious child. *Gbai* (tops) are the only playing things that are kept for any length of time.

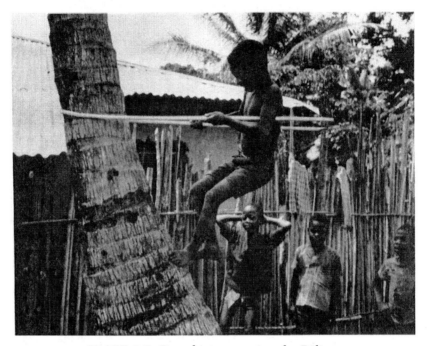

PLATE 5.5. Boy playing at using the *Baliŋ*.

In general, *Pele-seŋ* are highly valued and guarded by their young owners when they are new. Many fights break out over possession of a newly made or found toy. After a few days, when the newness wears off, the toy is passed from child to child, each of whom gets some enjoyment out of it. No toy has a long life because toys are treated rather roughly and interest in them quickly wanes.[12]

Boys occasionally build models of cars, houses, and kitchens but not of people or animals. One model of a rice kitchen was built on top of a termite mound on the farm and was quite accurate with a thatched roof, trapdoor, and so on. Another boy took great pains to build a wooden automobile, using splinters for nails. When he first began to "drive" (push) it around town, other boys gathered curiously to watch, but were not allowed to play with it. The next day, the boy relented and a few of his closer friends were driving it, but carefully. By the fourth day the car (now missing a wheel) was being driven and fought over by a large group of boys on the mother-ground, but the owner was nowhere in sight. By the end of a week, the car was lying broken and abandoned behind a house. I witnessed a similar sequence of events in the case of another boy who had captured a tortoise in the jungle.

Nsamenang (1992) sees considerable functional significance in children's toy construction: "Because it is not a West African tradition to provide children with toys, they are usually encouraged to create their own, making miniature replicas of common objects. . . . The genesis of the rich tradition of African sculpture, woodcuts, embroidery, leatherwork and pottery is rooted in this form of socialization" (p. 57).

THE FUNCTION OF MAKE-BELIEVE PLAY

Make-believe play can provide opportunities for children to acquire adult work habits and to rehearse social scenes. In many cases the transition from play work to real work is nearly seamless. However, some adult roles are just too complex to be acquired solely in the course of *Neé-pele*—blacksmithing, for example.

Let us compare, briefly, the blacksmith at work in his forge with children doing a make-believe recreation of blacksmithing. In the realm of social relations, the blacksmith enters into a number of reciprocal relationships: between himself and a helper, who may also be an apprentice; between himself and a client, for whom he makes a tool and from whom he exacts an obligation to work on his farm; and and between his wife or wives who take care of many of his needs in return for his protection and maintenance. In the make-believe play we see these social relationships duplicated. A boy of 8 or so is the blacksmith; two other boys of roughly the same age act as clients. A younger boy serves as helper, holding a "tool" for the "blacksmith" to "hammer" and fetching woodchips for the "fire." Finally, two girls, younger than 10, prepare and bring "food" for the smith to eat. The anvil is a rock and the tongs are a piece of bamboo that has been partially split along its length. Different types and sizes of sticks represent different hammers. The finished machete (a flat piece of wood) is given to its "owner," who goes off to cut brush with it.

The "blacksmith" and his co-actors use the appropriate language in carrying out their make-believe. The older boy is addressed as "smith" or "old man," the helper as "boy" or "son." The girls as "wife." The specialized blacksmith's tools and paraphernalia are also referred to by their proper names.

The blacksmith possesses complex technical skills, the most important of which is a basic understanding of metals and their reaction to various temperatures and stresses. Clearly, these technical skills are not acquired to any appreciable degree during make-believe play. The blacksmith is also an important ritual figure and will be called on to assist in administering oaths. I found no evidence to indicate that children were learning the ideological aspects of being a blacksmith through their play.

In reviewing the various examples I collected of children doing make-believe play, the learning of social relations appears to be paramount, especially such roles as *kuu* leader, husband, wife, elder, and chief, followed by learning language—especially symbols peculiar to the various occupational roles. One occasionally sees the beginnings of real skill learning, but ideology is apparently absent.

In some societies, make-believe play is considerably more elaborate than I observed (e.g., Wilson, 1963). In both Ghana and Central Africa, anthropologists have observed what amounts to a miniature society recreated by children (e.g., Centner, cited in Schwartzman, 1978). Goody (1992) reports on scaled down "kitchens" where 4- to 5-year-old girls pretend to grind grain using sand. Their rhythms and sung accompaniments also replicate adult patterns. Their 10-year-old sisters build small fires and cook soup in small pots. Brothers take the role of husband and, characteristically, criticize the consistency and flavoring of the soup. At 11 or so the girls offer their mothers assistance in the kitchen; by 13 they have full responsibility for preparing the family meal. Another charming example is provided by Margaret Read (1960): "A perennial amusement among Ngoni boys . . . was playing at law courts . . . In their high squeaky voices the little boys imitated their fathers whom they had seen in the courts, and they gave judgments, imposing heavy penalties, and keeping order in the court with ferocious severity" (p. 84).

Although Schwartzman (1978) cautions us that "children's behavior (particularly play behavior) does not always serve as a socializing and social ordering activity, as it may in fact be seen to challenge, reverse, and/or comment on and interpret the social order" (p. 25), in fact, make-believe play outside our own culture appears to be quite conservative. The following assessment of Mayan children at play is typical: "There is little elaboration or introduction of variation or complexity during the course of play. Scripts and roles are repeated over and over, almost ritualized" (Gaskins & Göncü, 1992, p. 32).

Parker's (1984) assessment of the role of make-believe is typical: "The ability to engage in make-believe games seems to be an adaptation for practicing domestic and extra-domestic subsistence tasks and associated sex-role differentiation" (p. 276). This frequent assertion that play affords children opportunities to practice skills[13] deserves some scrutiny, however:

> If practice or some form of training is necessary for the optimal development of skilled behavior, then we must ask . . . why practice *play*? Consider the alternatives. Practice outside of the play context might be extremely dangerous. If a young animal had to learn to fight during real fighting, it would be severely injured or killed. If it had to learn to hunt by hunting, it would starve. If it had to learn mothering by practicing on it's own offspring, it would have a poor reproduction record. . . . Furthermore, in all these "for real" contexts, arousal is liable to be very high, and it has been demonstrated experimentally that learning does not progress very well under conditions of high arousal.
>
> On the other hand, learning does not occur very well when arousal is too low, and most drill-type practice is boring. Similarly, teaching is boring and inefficient because it requires an investment by a second party, the teacher. Thus, while selection favors learning over instinct in many cases, it is unlikely to favor teaching or pure practice as educational media. This argument applies with equal force to *human* development as teaching and drill-type practice are conspicuously absent in most cultures. (Lancy, 1980b, p. 482, emphasis added).

What do adults think of children's make-believe play? Among the Kpelle, there is a feeling of mild tolerance—it is not as noisy and dangerous as other, more boisterous kinds of play. Erchak (1976/1977) mentions that one of a pair of twins is expected to become a *Ƶò*. The *Ƶò-na* observe the two as they mature, looking for signs of assertiveness. However, this is the only Kpelle case of which I am aware of adults scrutinizing children for their aptitude. Guatemalan peasants (Nerlove, Roberts, et al., 1974) apparently *do* pay attention to children's play. They make judgments about children's intelligence and initiative from observing them at play and assign them chores accordingly.

Of course, in our own society, we encourage children's symbolic play and support it through the purchase of dolls, rubber farm animals, puppets, and so on. We seek to influence our children's play quite deliberately in order to *push* and channel their development. As I found in my comparative study in Papua New Guinea (Lancy, 1983), there is one other type of society—maritime fishing and trading—that seems to push children intellectually as we do. The Wogeo are one such society (neighbors of the Ponamese whom I studied), and Hogbin (1970a) reports an episode of model canoe construction that is nearly unique in the annals of enculturation in terms of adults explicitly capitalizing on children's make-believe as an opportunity for instruction:

> Each lad makes a vessel for himself, and the party then adjourns to the shallow water off the beach. The men . . . sit watching and afterwards give a detailed commentary on the different craft taking part. This one . . . was unwieldy because the outrigger booms were too long, that one went crab-fashion because the float was crooked, the sail of a third was too small to take full advantage of the wind, and a fourth would have been more stable had a few stones been put into the hull. The patience of one man when his little son, too unskilled as yet to carve a model out of wood, had fashioned a rough craft from half a coconut shell, was most touching. He treated the boy's efforts with the utmost seriousness, and his criticism could hardly have been more carefully phrased if the canoe had been a masterpiece of ingenuity. Suggestions are usually put to the proof at once and additional information sought if a prediction fails to come true. (p. 143)

Do all societies foster rich opportunities for children's make-believe play? By no means. Some years ago I conducted a study (Lancy, 1982) in which I compared children in two American communities. In the one there was an array of adult work roles for the children to observe, and they did try them on through elaborate and varied make-believe play. In the other community, few adults were employed and children's play was correspondingly impoverished (see also Smilansky, 1978).

Another situation in which we might see only limited make-believe play occurs when children are expected to become self-sufficient from an early age. Hadza children, for example, are expected to forage on their own from as young as 3. Children as young as 5 can gather enough Baobab fruits to cover half their daily caloric needs. While in camp, they are given many chores: They are sent for wood and water, they care for infants, and they drive snakes from camp. There is little time for make-believe and adults do not act indulgently toward children's play (Blurton-Jones, 1993; see also LeVine & LeVine, 1963, on the Gusii of Kenya).

But, for the Kpelle, make-believe certainly is an important routine and its service in the enculturation of children is clear—at least to the outside observer. The relationship of children's *rule-governed* play or games to adult activity is much less apparent, notwithstanding the fact that the training or enculturating function of games is widely acknowledged in the theoretical writing of many developmental scholars. Vygotsky (1967) saw make-believe and games as reciprocal—the former as a fantasy world built on top of an implicit rule structure; the latter as governed by explicit rules but with an implicit fantasy or story at the core. In the next chapter we visit the mother-ground to observe children engaged in a sample of traditional games taken from the large stock found in Gbarngasuakwelle. Games are cataloged from an emic perspective. That is, I examine them within the indigenous category structure supplied by my Kpelle informants. But it is also necessary to examine these games from an etic perspective to assess their value as enculturative devices.

CHAPTER 6

Games and Models

We believe . . . that every society will be found to contain in its culture
certain autotelic folk models, with the help of which it socializes the
young.

—ANDERSON AND MOORE (1960, p. 207)

. . . society tries to provide a form of buffered learning through
which the child can make . . . step-by-step progress toward adult
behavior.

—ROBERTS AND SUTTON-SMITH (1962, p. 184)

Alan Anderson and Omar Khayyam Moore and Jack Roberts and Brian
Sutton-Smith were evidently all thinking along the same lines[1] regarding
the value of play—especially games—to children and society. Both pairs
of scholars stressed the routinized nature of these activities to enculturate
children. Games are enduring *artifacts*, a permanent part of a society's
repertoire, reused with each new generation. Both pairs also stressed the
sheltered quality of these learning opportunities. Children could risk "getting it wrong" without serious consequences. At the same time, from the
society's vantage point, games are clever devices—they are fun to play
("autotelic") and, thereby seduce the child into learning things society
thinks are important. Roberts and Sutton-Smith (1962) clearly demonstrate that the game inventory of any society tends to reflect and reinforce
the personal qualities and skills expected of successful adults in that society. In both theories the term "model" is used to imply that the game (or,
for Anderson and Moore, games, songs, folktales, etc.) somehow *abstracts*
essential *underlying* attributes from the culture and makes them available in
a form that is so attractive that children do not mind practicing them over
and over.

Vygotsky (1962, 1978) and Piaget (1965) also emphasized the sheltered learning aspect of play and games. Piaget, in studying children
learning to play marbles, demonstrated the gradual process whereby the

novice player comes to learn not only the rules of the game but rules qua rules. This study is described in a book titled *The Moral Judgement of the Child.* In his conversations with the young marble shooters, Piaget uncovered their nascent understanding of moral concepts like "fair versus unfair" and "cheating."

Although these theories are often invoked, there has been remarkably little research done that looks specifically at the enculturative function of games. There is, in fact, a curious bifurcation in the literature. Empirical studies of games and children's learning have almost all been done in the context of formal schooling (e.g., educational games or simulations), whereas studies (as opposed to lists or collections, which are legion) of naturally occurring games in culture have tended to focus exclusively on the more complex games played by adults such as Go or chess (Avedon & Sutton-Smith, 1971). The material in this chapter makes only a modest contribution to rectifying this scarcity. It does, however, reinforce these pioneering thinkers' key ideas.

DOING PLAY

It is an hour or so before nightfall. I have been copying the day's notes and need to stretch. As I come around a corner and into an open square, I surprise a group of six boys (between 5 and 11 years old) seated in a circle playing a game. They are very boisterous but, temporarily, my presence diverts their attention. They are playing a game classified as *Sua-kpé pele,* or hunting play, called *Saŋjao. Saŋjao* is the name of a large bird (hornbill sp.), and the game is called *Saŋjao, Woni-Kileé* (all birds). I have seen them play this game in mixed-sex groups numbering as many as eight. All players tap their fingers on the ground and sing a response to the leader's call. The leader begins:

> *Call:* "*Saŋjao.*"
> *Response:* "All birds!"
> *Call:* [Names another bird.]
> *Response:* "Leave it there forever."

The players continue tapping and singing until the leader names an animal that is not a bird and everyone must stop singing and tapping. If a player fails to stop, he is "beaten" and must drop out of the game. In fact, I notice that small children who fail to stop are often ignored or, at most, jostled. One youngster—a repeat offender—is sent away in tears, but he slips back into the circle after a short interval. On the other hand, older boys seem to deliberately and ostentatiously continue after an animal has been named and the game quickly descends into a bout of rough-and-tumble play. This chaos provides a nice opportunity for Kerkula—the apparent leader—to exert his authority in reestablishing order and the flow of the game. Kerkula comes in for quite a bit of taunting and there are calls of "You already named that one." "That's not a bird!" Were this in the United States, I would be appealed to as an adult to serve as the referee. But, here adults do not intervene in children's games.

Before I quite realize it, the group switches to *Menà-pu-kau* (put horn in the bowl), which is very similar. Here the leader names horned animals and the group responds, "*Bulu,*" which is the sound of the horn dropping in the bowl. If the leader names a nonhorned animal all must stop tapping and singing. This change sustains their interest for a bit more but, soon, the older boys get up and order their younger siblings to accompany them home. I collected three other games of this same type and they were quite popular—especially as darkness came on and when the play group spanned a wide age range (see Lancy, 1984)

One of the broadest categories of play for the Kpelle is *Pele-kee,* or, simply, "doing play." We would recognize most of the playforms in this category as games. Identifying them as models is not easy, however. The children themselves, of course, make poor informants as to the representational force or abstract meaning of a game, but adults are not much better. Interestingly, children rarely were even able to tell me the name of the game they were playing, so I had to turn to adult observers for this information.

A common ingredient in children's play is the loose sand lying everywhere. Children draw designs in the sand with sticks. They "build roads" by shuffling through the sand with their feet together, or with three fingers together. This is all called *Peliŋ-pele,* or drawing play, and the category also includes several games. Adults, when they want to show how something looks, freely draw in the sand, and it is clear that the sandy ground serves as a kind of outdoor "blackboard." Naturally, this type of play diminishes sharply during the rainy season when sloppy mud or hard-packed sand predominates.

Hiding is another prominent feature of many games, especially those included in the "hiding play" (*Loo-pele*) category, and one is tempted to link the pervasiveness of this skill in Kpelle games with the previously discussed emphasis on observation in children's acquisition of their culture.

Third, pebbles or seeds (*Koni-pele*, or stone play, which includes at least 10 distinct games) figure in well over half of all Kpelle games, and these games seem to implicate mnemonic, counting, and perceptual skills. Fourth, many games include call and response phrasing characteristic of Kpelle song (see Chapter 7), Again, my impression is that these games put a premium on memory and attention.

A final point is that games are stratified by age and gender. Most games are played by children only within a fairly narrow age range, and many of them are unisex. The first major category is *Sua-kpé pele*, or hunting play.

Sua-kpé pele takes up where *Neé-pele* (make-believe; see Chapter 5) leaves off. That is, it is founded on make-believe reenactments of specific adult activities (i.e., hunting) yet also has set rules and procedures for play. A limited number of elements from real-world hunting and bushwhacking are abstracted to create game features. This category includes a variety of play activities, two of which we have already discussed (e.g., *Saŋjao* and *Menà-pu-kau*). *Sua-pele* simulates group net hunting and is done in the town by a large group of 7- to 14-year-old boys. Ropes, representing "nets," are strung between buildings, and the boy designated as the "game" may not cross the ropes. He hides, other boys post themselves throughout the town, and the hunt leader tries to "flush out the game." When he has succeeded, he drives the game toward the nets and the other boys close in, throw the game to the ground, and "cut its throat." A variation takes place in the jungle when one boy is game and hides. Others try to find him and when one succeeds he calls loudly to the others to assist him.

In *Kpasa* (fighting), a younger member of the group of 6 to 12 boys, ages 10 to 14 is designated the "animal baby," and a second member is designated "animal mother." The other players attempt to "kill" (touch) the baby and if a player succeeds, he becomes the new mother. The mother tries to prevent this from happening by killing (touching) the "hunter." If the mother succeeds in touching a hunter four times (or one, two, or three times as determined by prior agreement) that player is out of the play. To start the plays, the mother says, "Throw it out!" The baby says, "Let's all go." The mother says, "I got you," when he touches a player. If it is the fourth touch, he says, "Go off." If, however, he loses count and fails to say "Go off" at the fourth touch (he may not touch a player several times in succession) the player starts again at zero. If a player manages to touch the baby, he says, "I have killed the *Kpasa* baby." The strategy of play appears to be for the hunters to spread out in a ring around the mother to draw him away and leave the baby unguarded.

Loma is the name of a type of antelope (probably *Cephalopholus—Duiker sp.*) as well as the name of a game. It is analogous to the Western game of "leapfrog." In *Loma*, eight or more boys, ages 8 to 12, line up and squat down on their haunches. The last player in the line "leapfrogs" each member in the line, then takes his place at the front of the line. A player who fails to make a leap is "out."

Boloŋ is a target made from a piece of the edoe or banana trunk, a papaya, or a stack of heavy leaves. The target is hung on a tree or stump and a line is drawn 8 to 25 feet away. One at a time, boys shoot an arrow at the target. The first person to hit the target collects and keeps all the arrows that were shot wide of the mark. Play continues until one person wins all the arrows.

Sua-iseler (wild animal) uses game animal symbolism but is categorized as *Loo-pele*, or hiding play (there are several other named hide-and-seek games). A group of boys or girls ages 10 to 12 meets before play begins and agrees on a "key" animal name. Then they gather in the mother-ground and invite others to play. Someone from the original group volunteers to go with an outsider to hide. Another outsider names a wild animal to the group leader. Then they call the member back from hiding; he is welcomed back by a chorus of "Wild animal, come let's shake hands. You come limping, did you meet up with any wild animals?" He answers, "Yes." "Did you meet animal *X*?" "Yes." Did it hurt you?" "No." This continues as the group leader asks him if he was hurt by a variety of animals, to all of which he answers, "No." Then the leader uses the key animal's name; again, the answer is no. Depending on the previously agreed on convention, the next animal (or the second, third, etc.) named after the key animal will be the one supplied by the outsider. To this animal the person being quizzed answers, "Yes."

These games model hunting, chasing prey, and bush lore, generally. Often played at night, or in the bush, they convey an air of danger, and the bush, with its wild animals, snakes, and forest spirits, is a dangerous place. Parker (1984) calls these agonistic exercise games. She provides a lengthy treatment, for example, of "aimed throwing," which shows gradual development in young males and is virtually absent in girls. This development has both cultural (e.g., games like *Boloŋ*) and biological components. For example, "at puberty . . . hormones stimulate specially primed cartilage cells in the shoulder. [However,] from early childhood boys have broader chests and longer forearms" (p. 278). These games also reveal, rather transparently, the relative quickness, cleverness, and status of the players. Nascent leaders among the children have ample opportunity to influence the direction and outcome of the game. By the same token, novice or less adept players are easily singled out. To this extent, then, these games serve the culture in imparting information to children and in establishing an incipient "pecking order."

Kweŋ are honey bees and this *Sua-kpé pele* is played by 10- to 14-year-old boys. Several march abreast with their arms over each other's shoulders. As they go along through the town they sing:

Call: "Bees."
Response: "Troublesome bees."

If they encounter anyone who refuses to move out of their path they split up and, singing *"Woooo"* (sound of bees), they attack the individual with blows. Interestingly, this playform closely parallels the actions of the *Poro Ẓò* and the Namu bush devil. When they see fit to do so, the *Poro* enter the town in force. All noninitiated women and boys (and anthropologists) are warned by a ringing bell to scurry for shelter inside their homes lest they inadvertently discover the identity of a masked figure or spy something they should not as the party of *Ẓò-na*, Namu, and initiated men moves through the town. The consequences for doing so are dire.

Peliŋ-pele (Drawing Play)

Peliŋ-pele, or drawing play, is distinguished by playforms in which geometric figures are drawn in the sand (Plate 6.1). *Pili* (jump) is exactly like the Western game of hopscotch but does not appear to have been recently introduced. The game is played by boys and girls ages 8 to 10. The squares are called towns and they are "captured" by the players. Figure 6.1, the diagram of the "towns," helps describe the sequence of play.[2]

A player begins at 1, throws a stone into square 2, then jumps over 2 to land with one foot in 3A, the other in 3B. Then he or she jumps to 4 on one foot, and to 5, turning in the air to face back to 1, then to 4 on one foot, to 3 with both feet, over 2 to 1. Then the player throws the stone in 3A and jumps as before, but now on one foot in 3B, avoiding 3A, and so it continues until he or she misses with the stone or in the jump, in which case a second player starts. If two players both succeed in this phase they continue to the "town capture" phase of the game. Players stand at 1 with their back to the diagram and throw the stone over their shoulder. If it lands in a square, they "own" it and for the remainder of the game only

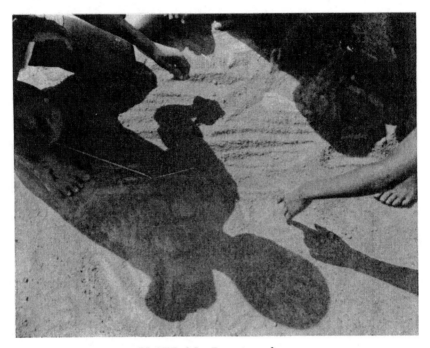

PLATE 6.1. Drawing play.

the "owner" is permitted to step in it. If he or she misses, the second player takes a turn. After the stone is thrown the player must jump as in phase one but now cannot step in any towns "owned" by an opponent. The game ends when all the towns are owned. Notice how the "text" of this game harkens back to the period in Kpelle history when intervillage hostilities were rife in much the same way that contemporary English children's play reflects events and ideas dating from medieval times (Opie & Opie, 1969).

Ma-mauŋ (name of a bush)-*kau* (seed) is another drawing game. The *Ma-mauŋ* seed, which is round, hard, and about 1 centimeter in diameter, is "shot" in a manner quite similar to marbles. A circle is drawn on the

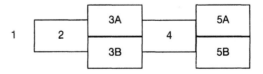

FIGURE 6.1. Diagram of *Pili* game.

ground and arms are attached to it at equal distances. All players have their own arm and place their seed at the end of the arm. They shoot the seed in the direction of the next player's arm (moving clockwise). If the seed lands on the arm, neither short of it nor beyond, shooters get to extend their arm by the distance from the arm to the perimeter of the circle. This continues until one player's arm crosses the next player's and the game is won. The size of the circle and the number of arms varies with the number of players, but three players with a 20-centimeter-diameter circle is a minimum. A three-player game might look like the illustration in Figure 6.2.

A variation on *Ma-mauŋ-kau* is *Maniŋ*, which is a shortened form of Mandingo, indicating that the game was introduced by the Mandingo people. Here an equal-armed cross is used with two to four players, each one starting at one end of an arm. The cross is drawn deeply in the sand creating "tracks." One boy pokes/shoots his *Ma-mauŋ* seed with his index finger laid flat on the ground toward the center of the cross. If the seed stays in the track and rolls across the center, the shooter measures the distance from the point at which it stopped to the center and adds the length to his arm. Thus when it is his turn to shoot again he will be shooting from further away. Each player gets one shot per turn and the game continues until one player has successfully shot his seed across the center four times.

Koni-kee Pele (Stone Play)

As with sand, stones are the "building blocks" of play. Infants, when they are permitted to crawl along the ground, discover stones and convert them into playthings. The infant picks up a stone, tastes it, looks at it, throws it,

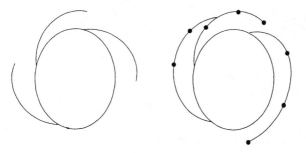

FIGURE 6.2. Diagram of *Ma-mauŋ-kau* game.

crawls to it, picks it up, and repeats the sequence ad infinitum. Stones are used extensively in *Neé-pele* as money, snails, peppers in a stew, and so on. Stones are used as ammunition in slings and slingshots and thrown at dogs and goats for sport. Finally, stones are used in the games listed under *Koni-kee pele,* or stone play (Plate 6.2). For example, this category includes the games *Koni-soo, Loa-koo,* and *Kpili-gelee* which all involve *throwing* stones and resemble *bocce, petanques,* or pitching pennies.

On an evening when there is no moonlight, a family will gather around the fire inside their house, passing the time in conversation and play. They may well be playing *Doo-nyeé* (put in the hand). In *Doo-nyeé,* there are two sides each with two to four players. One player will take a stone and pretend to place it in his or her own and in each of his or her teammates' clenched fists. The stone has been placed in one of the four to eight fists and it is now the turn of a member of the opposing team to guess which hand it is in. The player takes each fist in his or her own hands, saying, "*Bem*" (just a sound), and finally decides. If the player guesses wrong, the team members who have clenched fists advance one step in making their rice farm. If the player is correct, *his or her* team may advance

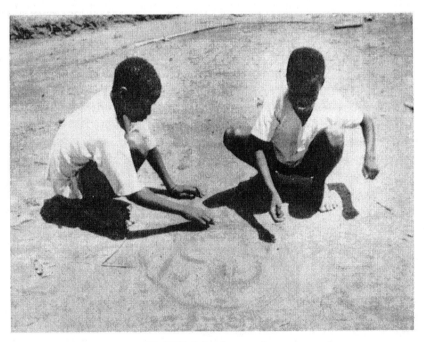

PLATE 6.2. Stone play.

a step. I use the expression "advance a step" because this game is exactly analogous to many Western board games with dice. Each team takes turns hiding the stone and the number of steps varies with the interest and enthusiasm of the players; the steps in the rice cycle can be broken down almost infinitely.

Some of the possible steps are listed below:

1. You start farm.
2. You cut brush.
3. You cut trees.
4. Farm dies out.
5. You get bamboo sticks out so they don't burn.
6. You carry fire to farm.
7. You burn the land.
8. The rain washes the ashes away.
9. You clear remaining, unburnt sticks.
10. Wife starts planting and scratching.
11. Wife finishes planting and scratching.
12. The rice comes up.
13. Rice grows up.
14. The grain appears.
15. The grain is exposed.
16. The grain ripens.
17. The first stalk is cut.
18. You carry it to the kitchen.
19. You beat it.
20. You offer some to the ancestors.
21. You cut the remaining rice.
22. The man builds the scaffold.
23. You put the rice on the scaffold.
24. He cuts the sticks for kitchen.
25. He carries them to farm.
26. He builds your kitchen.
27. You make your mats.
28. You put mats in loft of kitchen.
29. You put rice in loft.
30. You lock up the kitchen.
31. You call bees, snakes and leopard to guard your kitchen (i.e., from your opponents in the game, who, because their farm is not finished,will want to take your rice).
32. End of game.

Besides the fact that *Doo-nyeé* is fun and will be played for its own sake, it teaches four important lessons to children. First, it familiarizes them with the elements of rice farming[3] and, more important, its step or chainlike character. Second, it mirrors the group work nature of rice farming in that it is played by teams rather than single players. Third, the two teams, like neighboring farms, will advance at about the same rate because, being a game of pure chance, each team is equally likely to guess correctly. Fourth, the chance factor in the game is also present in rice farming. Many elements are beyond one's control, such as the weather, pests, and unreliable kuu members.

Nyinaŋ (bad spirit) is usually played by girls ages 10 to 14 at night on the mother-ground. Although it is another example of stone play, functionally, it is similar to the boy's animal-naming games described earlier. The girls sit on the ground in a circle with their feet flat on the ground, A lappa is draped over their knees. One girl sits in the middle as the girls in the circle pass a stone under their knees around the circle. The girl in the center must try to guess the location of the stone at any given moment. When the girl discovers the stone she must fight the person holding it to wrench it from her grasp. If she succeeds in grasping the stone, she joins the circle and the girl who gave it up now takes her place in the center. Meanwhile, songs accompany the play.

Too-too is a stone game played by young boys and girls (ages 6 to 9) and may be considered training for the more complex stone games discussed later. Thirty-three stones are arranged in a line, which may be straight but is more often curved or crooked. The player must touch each stone and say, "*Too*," for all 33 stones in order, at a high rate of speed. At the end of a successful runthrough, one stone is taken away and put in the player's pile. The player then starts over again and continues in this fashion until he or she misses a touch or a *Too*, then the other player starts. *Tiaŋ-kai-sii* adds new elements to *Too-too*. The stones number 10 to 25 and are arranged in a straight line. Players must hold their breath as they touch each stone and say, "*Tiaŋ-kai-sii taang*" (one), "*Tiaŋ-kai-sii verre*" (two), and so on, to 10 or 25. The game coincides with the child learning to count and manipulate numbers.

Closely related to stone-counting games are *Kpa-keleŋ-je* and *Kwa-tinaŋ*. *Kpa-keleŋ-je* (no, continue) is played by both sexes, ages 8 to 15. Ten stones are placed in a line. One player points to the first stone and says, "Is this the one?" The other player, whose back is turned, says, "Yes, if you miss the rock, you'll break your thigh." The first player again points to the rock and says, "Is this the one?" Second player answers, "No, continue." The first player then points to the second stone and asks the question. This time the answer is "Yes." Then he points to the first stone, answer, "No"; second stone, answer, "No"; then the third stone, and the answer should be, "Yes"; and so on for all the stones. The player must then have a mental map of the stones and follow the pointing in his or her imagination. If he or she misses, the players switch places. This game, then, is similar to the "old man spider game" and is a foretaste of the more difficult game, *Kwa-tinaŋ* (we have turned around).

Kwa-tinaŋ is played by older children and, occasionally, adults. Again there are two players, one to point at the stones, another to call directions. The stones are laid out as in Figure 6.3.

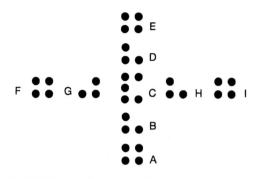

FIGURE 6.3. Diagram of *Kwa-tinaŋ* game.

Starting from A, the player whose back is turned says:

"Take from four." (The other player takes one stone away from A.)
"Take from three." (The other player takes a stone from B.)
"Take from five." (Stone taken from C.)
"Take from three." (Stone taken from D.)
"Take from four." (Stone taken from E.)
"Now we turn around."
"Take from four." (Stone taken from F.)
"Take from three." (Stone taken from G.)
"Take from four." (Stone taken from C.)
"Take from three." (Stone taken from H.)
"Take from four." (Stone taken from I.)
"Now we turn around."
"Take from three." (Stone taken from A.) Etc.

Play continues until the player calling directions makes a mistake and then the players switch places, or until he or she gets through all the stones without a mistake. In a small experiment, I had boys attempt to complete the *Kwa-tinaŋ* under controlled conditions. I found considerable evidence of a developmental pattern. Younger boys seemed to memorize each configuration because on each trial they proceeded a little further (there are 47 moves, counting "We have turned around"). Older boys showed signs of acquiring a mental map of the stones because they advanced in large jumps from try to try.

Kwa-tinaŋ, Too-too, Tiaŋ-kai-sii and *Kpa-keleŋ-je* are all counting games and an important aspect of each is "place keeping." Place keeping means the ability to hold numbers or places in one's head. In a society that lacks writing, arithmetic must be largely performed mentally (Gay & Cole, 1967), although people do occasionally use piles of stones to aid their place keeping. It seemed reasonable to believe that these games function as routines to develop counting skills. Part confirmation came from interviews with informants on the subject of how children learn to handle numbers. A father will tell his child, "Go into the house and fetch two bananas." If he brings the incorrect number, he is told to go back and try again. If he succeeds, he then may be told, "Go now and bring four Kola nuts from your mother," and so on. *Tiaŋ-kai-sii* was specifically mentioned in this discussion as teaching children number–names.

Koni-peniŋ (Stone Magic)

I would like to turn now to *Koni-peniŋ*, or stone magic. I collected five examples of this genre of play, which is practiced exclusively by boys over 15. One of these is *Meni-ka-ɣenye* which means, "There is something in the world." Two boys play it (or "demonstrate" might be a better word) and the stones are arranged in five piles, as indicated in Figure 6.4. The first player says, "There is something in the world," and takes two stones from A (quickly). The second player then says, "There is nothing in the world," and takes the remaining stones from A. This sequence is repeated for piles B, D, and E. Then player one says, "You say there is nothing in the world—take two stones from this pile" (C). Player two does as he is told. Player one takes the remaining three stones from C, then says, "You say there's nothing in the world so I will take from you the two stones you just took." Then the two players begin reconstructing the original piles, A, B, D, and E, but this time they each build two piles from the stones in their hands rather than combining them. This, of course, exhausts the six stones that player two has collected. Then player one puts three stones in C, then adds his two remaining stones, saying, "And here are the two stones I took from you." I use the term "demonstration" to describe *Meni-ka-ɣenye* because it is not truly a game even though it appears that one player has gained a two-stone advantage. Actually, both players have to

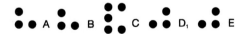

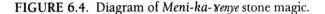

FIGURE 6.4. Diagram of *Meni-ka-ɣenye* stone magic.

cooperate to "fool" an audience. Fooling the audience is the essence of stone magic. The audience is not expected to be able to solve the "problem." Boys who know *Koni-peniŋ* put up a show of resistance when asked to perform and they refuse to divulge their "secrets" except for a fee.

Bambé is played by boys in their mid- to late teens. Although not stone magic per se, it shares this "fooling the uninitiated" theme. *Bambé* means "perception" and the object of play is for initiated players to learn to perceive "signs," which the uninitiated cannot perceive. *Bambé* is also the name of the secret society in which the signs are taught.[4] It has a *Ẓ̀o*, a boy approximately age 18. Membership is restricted to males and if a boy wishes to join he must first bring some gifts such as dried rats, birds, or fish, some rice or palm oil. The *Ẓ̀o* prepares these foods and serves them to the members. After the food is eaten, the new initiate is told the secrets of the society and also told that if he divulges them he will be fined.

The *Ẓ̀o* leads his group to the mother-ground—it is about 7 P.M. on a moonlit evening (Plate 6.3). Sitting in a semicircle on the veranda of a house, they begin singing and beating a small drum. Gradually, an audience of girls and boys and young adults gathers and the *Ẓ̀o* calls out, "We

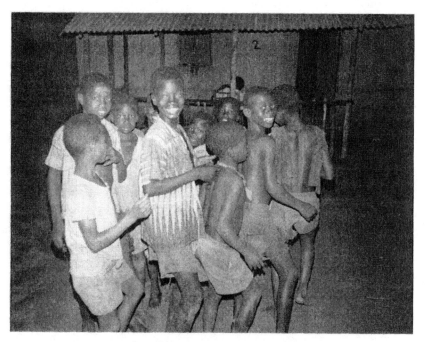

PLATE 6.3. Boys preparing to do *Bambé*.

have medicine to find lost things, come try it." A young man in the audience comes forward, amid much teasing and tittering, and agrees to hide some small item. Before he does he picks a boy from among the *Bambé* society members and sends him away so that he cannot see where the item has been hidden. This boy then returns and accepts a small weed stalk from the *Zò*. He then proceeds to touch people and likely hiding places— in corners, under stools—each time bringing it to his nose to detect the "smell" of the hidden item. Actually, he is attending to signs given by the *Zò* and the members that tell him when he is getting close. As long as the sign is displayed he knows he is getting closer. When it goes off he knows he is moving away from the hidden item. There are a number of signs which can be used, such as the *Zò* folding his arms across his chest, crossing his legs, or scratching his head. The drummer may increase the tempo or the singers may increase the volume of their singing. When he has located the item, he continues sniffing around and then comes back to the location or person on whom the item has been hidden. There is much opportunity for ribaldry on the part of both hider and finder. Older boys seem more willing to use this occasion to "ham it up." There are parallels here with such phenomenon as the potlatch, where Kwakiutl women mock the bombastic behavior of chiefs (Codere, 1956). Younger *Bambé* members, on the other hand, tend to be very serious lest they miss the sign. The signs are continually varied so that the audience cannot guess what they are. Each member takes a turn at playing sleuth, and this continues until they lose their audience.

I asked Yelɛkɛ and other informants why a boy should join the *Bambé* secret society. He replied that this was necessary so that the boy would learn to recognize signs. If a boy is a member of *Bambé*, he will be able to come into the house and notice immediately whether anything is missing and then quickly call, "Thief, thief," so that the rogue may be caught. Otherwise he will not notice anything. The boy should also be able to recognize more formal signs (*Tau*):

1. Pissava palm fibers hanging over a fence means "keep out."
2. Rope across a path with leaves hanging from it means "danger."
3. If you are on a *kuu* (cooperative work group; see Chapter 4) and the group has left the town without you, you follow them. If you come to a branch in the path, the wrong path will be covered with leaves.
4. A pile of rice on a leaf on the path to a farm is a sign the owner has made a sacrifice to his ancestors.

Other signs are used to direct a hunting party to game, advise a friend that he is in trouble, and so on.

Bambé is interesting in another respect. Because it had not been played in the town for at least 10 years, I had to "teach" it to a new group of boys.[5] I appointed an older boy as *Zö* and then, with 14 boys chosen randomly from all boys ages 8 to 13 presently living in the town, taught them the signs. They eagerly participated and easily fell into the secret nature of the play. Other boys who were not part of the group begged to learn to play and even spied on the teaching sessions, so a "guard" had to be posted. Adults clearly remembered how it was played and treated it as a significant element in the enculturation of youth. Yet, they seemed incapable of dealing with the reality of *Bambé*'s apparent demise. Again, we see the paradox of play (Lancy, 1980b). Having children learn something about signs is clearly valued, but outright teaching of signs, where learning is coerced, is not. So, a convenient playform gets the job done. But, play *must* be voluntary; hence, children can choose not to play *Bambé* and a valued cultural routine for children's development is lost to the society.

DEVELOPMENTAL TRENDS IN GAME PLAY

Piaget (1951) identifies three types of games: practice games, symbolic games, and games with rules. These predominate in age ranges from 0 to 18 months, 2 to 6 years, and 7 to 11 years, respectively. The practice game involves the deliberate repetition of a particular action, such as throwing, pushing, picking up, and so on. This repetition is apparently enjoyable as an end in itself. The young child enjoys exercising his newly emerging sensorimotor powers.

I witnessed few of these practice games in very young children. Two factors seem to account for this absence. First, infants are kept rather severely confined for the first 2 years of life; when awake they are almost inevitably found either at the teat or wrapped tightly onto someone's back. Second, when they are left free to roam, they do so in the company of children 3 to 4 years older and these children invariably "play with" the infants constantly. Specifically, the infants are given roles to play as babies in the make-believe play of older children. Given a chance, babies happily indulge in practice games. I frequently played games with one child of about 13 months. He alternately put a small can on his head and on my head, knocked it off, picked it up, rolled it, and hit it.

Piaget's symbolic games correspond perfectly with *Neé-pele*, or make-believe, but the symbolic games of children in Gbarngasuakwelle do not appear to have the range that Piaget found among his subjects. There appears to be little fantasizing with the supernatural, for example; rather, the symbols appear to be drawn entirely from the real world and tend to represent adult work activities almost exclusively. Older children, however, do learn and interact with a rich store of supernatural figures when they begin listening to and telling stories at about 8 years of age (see Chapter 7). As Piaget discovered, symbolic games shade into games with rules, such as *Pili* and *Geleŋ* (Lancy, 1975a), which involve "capturing towns." Other games, such as *Neni-polo*, "old man spider," and *Kpasa*, are full of symbolism, and *Sua-kpé pele*, or hunting play, might be called symbolic games with rules. Turning to games with rules, we see that there are several that require intense concentration. We might label these "paying attention" or "discrimination" games (cf. Roth, cited in Schwartzman, 1978, p. 75) and they include the games in which players must remember the configuration of stones when their back is turned, animal-naming and stone-hiding games, and, of course, *Bambé*. On the other hand, with the exception of *Malaŋ*, discussed in the next section, there are no games that demand "strategic" skills.[6] Nor are there many games that call for such physical skills as running, jumping, throwing, and catching. The only physical skill that is called for is throwing or shooting small stones or seeds.[7]

The amount of time that a child has to devote to game playing peaks at about age 7. Prior to that time the child is closely confined, and after age 7, the child becomes an integral member of the family working unit. This means that, relatively speaking, make-believe and the simpler games predominate. Girls are less likely to play games of any kind than are boys. Also, consistent with research done in the United States (Lever, 1978), games played exclusively by boys tend to be more complex than those played exclusively by girls or by both sexes. This does not stem from a lack of aptitude or interest but, rather, from a lack of time. Women work longer hours than men, and girls, until the age of 14 or so, stay pretty close to their mothers. The nature of women's work is such that many tasks are simple enough and do not demand great strength. Thus, certain tasks fall naturally to the young girl, such as taking care of infants, sweeping the house, cooking, weeding, and so on. Men's work, on the whole, is more complex and demands greater strength or physical dexterity. Therefore, boys begin adult work at a later age, leaving them more time to play.

Table 6.1 presents an age-by-playform matrix that shows the percentage of children at each age (within the range selected for this project) in Gbarngasuakwelle who said they could play a particular game. The table shows a clear developmental progression. By age 6 already, half the sample have mastered the very elementary games *Too-too* and *Gbini*. By contrast, *Kpa-keleŋ-je*, *Nyinaŋ*, *Pili*, and *Ma-mauŋ-kau* would seem to form a natural set of more complex games that are not played much before age 8. Similarly, the last four games in Table 6.1 begin to appear in the average child's repertoire no earlier than age 10 or 11. These last four are not more complex than the previous four but do require certain physical skills that very young children may lack.

There is an apparent attenuation in mastery of many of the more complex games as shown in the lower third of the table. This can be accounted for by three factors. First, my study concentrated on preadolescence so I have fewer data for play among children older than 13. Second, from my interviews, I deduced that, just as the more complex work skills are acquired by only a fraction of the eligible population (see Table 8.1),

TABLE 6.1. Percentage of Children Able to Play Selected Games

Games	Age (yr)							
	6	7	8	9	10	11	12	13
Too-too	52	91	85	97	96	90	95	100
Gbini	52	67	71	76	87	84	74	91
Saŋ-jao	24	57	68	90	83	68	74	91
Too-kiki-ya	24	43	62	72	74	84	84	73
Kpa-keleŋ-je	4	10	24	45	52	42	63	82
Nyinaŋ	4	14	27	45	44	74	74	64
Pili	4	14	21	55	39	63	53	64
Ma-mauŋ-kau	8	10	21	62	44	53	47	55
Sua-iseler	4	5	3	3	9	21	26	18
Kwa-tinaŋ	0	0	6	10	9	16	21	18
Old man spider	0	0	3	10	9	16	21	9
Kpasa	0	0	3	0	13	21	16	18

complex playforms are not learned by everyone. Third, older boys seem receptive to introduced playforms and these displace the traditional Kpelle games, as I show in Chapter 10.

All the games cited in the table have rules and learning the rules appears to be a crucial aspect of learning to play. Several anecdotes reveal the difference between "knowing the rules" and "following the rules." I watched two boys, one age 10, another age 8, attempting to play *Mamauŋ-kau*. The older boy meticulously drew the circle, then drew his arm. The younger boy began drawing an arm at the circumference of the circle but drew it improperly. It was too long and curved in the wrong direction. The older boy erased the improperly drawn arm and drew a correct one. Then he took his turn shooting the seed. As he was shooting, however, the other boy was adding to his own arm by drawing a crooked tail on it. The older boy looked at the embellishment and said, "You don't know anything," and walked away in disgust.[8] On another occasion, four boys gathered to play *Blee*. The first boy to try his luck in finding the ring searched around in the sandpile with his finger instead of making a single jab or cut with a stick. He was admonished for this error. The pile was reformed and the ring hidden, and he was permitted to try again. He followed the rule this time although he did not find the ring. He continued to play.

These two examples illustrate that before a child may participate in a multiplayer game, he must have at least a basic understanding of the rules of play. He may make a mistake, he may be unskilled in his play, and for this he will be teased or lightly slapped. If, however, he does not know the rules or the structure of the play, he is not permitted to play at all. No one takes the time to teach him the rules. The principal reason that learning to play a game must somehow be accomplished before one actually plays it is that virtually all games are played rapidly. One afternoon, I watched a group of boys play *Loma, Bulo, Goli-tuaŋ,* and *Meyuŋ* all in the space of 20 minutes. During this time the boys were constantly talking and moving except when the rules called for them to be still. There was no transitional discussion or argument as the group switched from one game to the next.

Malaŋ is also played with great speed. Although boys were somewhat tolerant of my attempts to learn to play, adult informants continually demanded that I make a move before I had analyzed the situation and was "ready." *Kwa-tinaŋ* illustrates a game in which knowing the rules and following the rules are clearly distinct. To play, one must understand that on each move, it is necessary to guess the number of stones in a pile and use the correct number in the phrase "Take one from _____." One must also learn that after every five piles, one "turns around" and travels along the other arm of the cross. These are the rules or the structure of play. Following the rules requires storing a mental map of the piles so that one remembers what the piles looked like initially and how they have changed with each succeeding turn. In trials I conducted with *Kwa-tinaŋ*, younger boys got hung-up with the structure of play. They had difficulty in remembering the phrases "take one from" and "turn around." Older boys had no such difficulty. For example, older boys might say, "Take from three . . . No! . . . Take from two," indicating that they knew what was required but had difficulty in searching through memory. Younger boys did not do this but were apt to ask a question such as, "Do we turn around yet?"

How then do children learn the rules of a game? Whenever a group of children gather to play, younger children are present as spectators. The gap in age between spectator and player is never very great so that 4-year-olds watch 6-year-olds and 8-year-olds watch 10-year-olds. This observation by young spectators is often followed by imitation. Two circles of five observed a group of older children playing *Pili* (hopscotch). When the older children leave, the girls take over the *Pili* drawing and jump up and down and in and out of the squares. Clearly, a great deal is learned about game rules from watching them being played. *Bambé, Sua-iseler,* and *Koni-peniŋ* are exceptions. In these playforms the rules are not easily learned by inspection. In fact, it is this mystery feature that makes them exciting. Thus, learning the rules requires that they be taught by someone who knows them.

Some games possess similar structures and can be grouped into sets. *Too-too, Kpa-keleŋ-je,* and *Kwa-tinaŋ* form one such set. *Loo-paye-paye, Gbini,* and *Geleŋ* form another set and so on. It seems likely that, since members of the set have similar structures, a child might learn the rules of *Kwa-tinaŋ.* more easily if he has already mastered *Too-too* and *Kpa-keleŋ-je.* Proof of this hypothesis would require extensive experimentation or a longitudinal study, neither of which was done. The results in Table 6.1 are suggestive, however. At age 7, 91% of the children indicated they could play *Too-too,* 10% of the children can play *Kpa-peleŋ-je,* and 0% play *Kwa-tinaŋ.* At age 10, the figures are 96%, 52%, and 9%, respectively. At 13, the figures are 100%, 82%, and 18%. Approaching these data from a slightly different perspective, we find that 100% of those who knew how to play *Kpa-keleŋ-je* also listed *Too-too* as one of the games they played. Of those who could play *Kwa-tinaŋ,* 100% knew how to play *Too-too* and 90% knew how to play *Kwa-keleŋ-je.*[9]

In the next section, we consider a very special seed game—one played primarily by adult men.

MALAŊ AND SHOWING SENSE

Malaŋ is the Kpelle version of a game that Culin (cited in Avedon & Sutton-Smith, 1971) has called "the national game of Africa" (p. 94) *Malaŋ* is the seed used in the game, A "gameboard," called *Kpeleŋ*, is placed between two players. There are six cup-shaped depressions on each side of the board, and one at each end for holding the captured seeds of the two players, respectively. Four seeds are placed in each of the 12 cups. One player begins by taking all the seeds from a cup on his side and dropping them, one at a time, into the cups to the right. He continues dropping the seeds into the cup, including those on his opponent's side, always moving counterclockwise, until there are none left in his hand. Then it is the other player's turn. If the last seed lands in a cup on the opponent's side that previously had one or two seeds in it, making a total of two or three, he may capture these seeds and place them in the "capture cup" on his right. The game is over when one player has no more seeds on his side to move, and the winner is the player who has captured the most seeds. Lancy (1975a) presents a lengthier description with variations.

The key to winning at *Malaŋ* is to plan a strategy of moves (see also Cole et al., 1971, pp. 182–184) well in advance, which helps to explain why players can make their moves so quickly. At the same time, one must anticipate the opponent's moves by figuring out what his strategy will be. This ability to anticipate a variety of seed/cup configurations requires the kind of shifting mental map that is also essential in *Kwa-tinaŋ*. In a miniexperiment, I tested five older men who were good at *Malaŋ* on their ability to do *Kwa-tinaŋ* None took longer than two trials to complete the problem. Figure 6.5 diagrams one *Malaŋ* strategy.

After perhaps 10 to 20 moves, during which a strategist has laid a trap for his opponent, the board looks like the diagram in Figure 6.5. The strategist is the player on the bottom who has maneuvered so that his opponent has no seeds on his side. Meanwhile, the strategist has collected a prefigured number of seeds in each of his six cups, seven in the cup on the far left, six in the next, and so on. It is the strategist's move. He moves his

a = 0	b = 0	c = 0	d = 0	e = 0	f = 0
A = 7	B = 6	C = 5	D = 4	E = 3	F = 1

FIGURE 6.5. Diagram of *Malaŋ* strategy.

seed from F to f. The opponent has only one choice, he must move the single seed from f to e. Then the strategist moves the seeds in E. At the end of his move there are two seeds in e and one in f; he captures the two in e, leaving the one in f. The opponent again has only one move—f to e. The strategist now moves the seeds from D and again captures two seeds. This will continue as, in six moves, the strategist captures 10 seeds to his opponent's 0.

There are no *Malaŋ* tournaments per se, but a kind of "round robin" does take place. A man will bring out his board and will challenge another to play. A group of men quickly gathers to watch and one will put in a request to "play the winner." The winner of the first match will play this newcomer and so it goes, each man continuing to play if he wins or relinquishing his place if he loses. Most adult men know how to play, but skill level varies enormously and, in practice, a man is unlikely to offer to play the winner unless his skill is roughly equivalent to those already playing.

In talking to my informants, I asked the question "Why should a boy learn *Malaŋ*?" The answer was "To learn respect for the old people." *Malaŋ* is learned neither easily nor quickly, and as a boy is repeatedly beaten by his older teacher, or reprimanded for his stupid play, he can not help but develop a healthy respect for the better player. My informants claimed that this respect is pervasive so that a young man will lack respect for his elders if he has not learned to play *Malaŋ*. By the same token, I never observed girls or women playing the game. Indeed, Zaslavsky (1973), reviewing studies of the game in other parts of Africa, notes, "Young girls were warned that their breasts would not develop, and no men would marry them [if they played the game]. Thus the men were assured that the game would not distract the women and girls from their assigned chores in the field and the home" (p. 124)

Readers must realize, however, that the most demanding use of mathematics in this society occurs in the game of *Malaŋ*. There is no other activity that requires the degree of complex place keeping, addition, subtraction, and division skills as *Malaŋ*. For example, in one version of the game, a player may elect to scoop the seeds out of one cup on his side and keep them in his hand on several successive turns. Then, when the opportunity is right, he will play out all the seeds from his hand. He can not count the seeds in his hand without his opponent seeing and counting them too, so he has to keep a running record in his head of how many seeds there are in his hand. Furthermore, he must be able to determine, at a glance, how the outcome will look after he has distributed the seeds. The strategy could easily backfire if the last seed landed on his side of the board. Earlier, I identified a game set consisting of *Too-too, Kpa-keleŋ-je,* and *Kwa-tinaŋ* and the evidence suggested that learning each game helped prepare one for the next, more complex one, in the set. I believe that this set, taken as whole, teaches many of the skills that are combined in *Malaŋ,* and, in fact, that *Malaŋ* might be added to the set as its most complex member.

At one time, my informants told me, you could tell how powerful a man was by his *Malaŋ* board. A "skilled player . . . may . . . be celebrated in song" (Zaslavsky, 1973, p. 124). A chief would not only own a very large one, but it would be finely made with human, animal, abstract, and *Poro*-inspired motifs as carved decoration. Boys, even those who had learned to play, did not own boards or even simple replicas. *Malaŋ* symbolizes the subordinate status of young men to older men.

A boy typically learns to play *Malaŋ* from his father or grandfather. He will have watched the game being played many times and will have learned the rules. He will "beg" his father or grandfather to teach him the game. If the paternal figure consents to do this, he will employ one of three "teaching methods." The most common is simply for the boy and older man to play together. The older man will say, "Now, pay attention to how I play and you will learn it." If the boy makes a good move or employs a successful strategy his teacher does not congratulate him per se but, rather makes an exaggerated show of displeasure at the losses he has suffered. When the boy makes a poor move, his teacher pounces and distributes his seeds and takes the captured seeds with obvious relish, saying, "You see where your foolish play has brought you?"

Because of the disparity in skill, however, it requires considerable patience for an older man to play with a boy. Therefore, some men prefer to "coach" a son or grandson who is playing against one of his peers. This can be done in one of two ways. The "coach" may tell his pupil how to make each single move. He will say, "Play from one," or "Play from four," indicating the cup (from one to six running from left to right) from which the boy should distribute the seeds. Here the coach works out his strategies and the boy learns the strategies from having to carry them out. The second way requires the coach only to comment on the moves as the boy makes them or attempts to make them. The following remarks are a sampling of Yelɛkɛ's directions to his son as he was teaching him to play *Malaŋ*:

> "You have the same number of seeds [i.e., both players], if you try hard you will win some."

"Don't play that one, put one here [points to cup]."

"If you give all your seeds out what will you play with?"

"Play it, you will capture three cups."

"You have spoiled it, if you play like that you won't win any."

"Look in this cup, if there are four seeds in it, you'll capture two cups, if there are five, you capture one."

"No, it is his turn to play, you can't play two times in a row."

"If you can win by playing the seeds from the fifth cup, then play them. Aren't there five seeds in there? OK, play from there . . . you see!?"

The teacher assumes his pupil knows the rules. He may tolerate an occasional lapse, as when the boy tries to make two moves in succession, but, as I found out, he has too little patience to train a complete novice. The teacher can teach short-range strategy but does not teach long-range strategy. In the teaching situation I have described, Yɛlɛkɛ would comment on each individual move and could justify his advice in terms of the immediate consequences of each move, but he did not attempt to assist the boy in planning long-range strategy. These long-range strategies do exist and the outsider can discern and record them (Lancy, 1975a), but players cannot articulate them. I succeeded in conveying to my research assistant that I wanted to learn such strategies. He had no trouble demonstrating the moves, but he could not verbalize them in either Kpelle or English, nor could he verbalize any general rules for "good" strategies or "bad" strategies

Thus, *Malaŋ* is apparently learned in much the same way that complex skills such as weaving, leatherwork, and blacksmithing are learned, and knowing how to play *Malaŋ* is one of the compelling attributes of manhood. Most of these findings have been replicated and extended by Jean Retschitzki (1990) in his comprehensive study of the Baoulé version of this game as reported in *Stratégies des jouers d'Awélé*. His study emphasizes the tremendous skill an accomplished player must have because there are a "multiplicité des variants . . ." (p. 31) and because even simple versions allow for a great number of possible strategies. His work is particularly valuable because he was able to identify unique stages in the development of expert players. For example, boys of about 15 are quite adept at utilizing various offensive strategies but still tend to display weak defensive tactics. Although improved memory for board configuration patterns is undoubtedly part of this developmental process, Retschitzki (1989) estimates that there are 10^{12} possible configurations—far too many to hold in memory. Instead, he sees success depending on the use of powerful heuristics and hypotheticodeductive reasoning.

James Gibbs (1965/1988), one of the principal students of the Kpelle, has described their ethos:

> Kpelle culture has two conflicting dominant themes. The first is a stress on personal autonomy and individual achievement of status . . . the basic quest is for the individual acquisition of wealth through hard work and shrewd investment of this wealth in persons. At advantageous times one collects the social debts thus created. Throughout there is not too subtle a stress on the instrumental manipulation of others to one's own advantage. What is significant is that this is an individual enterprise, not one of a corporate group. However, if a man is prudent, he will not neglect his supernatural resources. He will protect and enhance his gains by investing in medicines and charms to hold his wives and protect his crops; perhaps he will use sorcery to slow the progress of his rivals. . . . The counterweight to this theme of individual advancement is the stress on conformity and regulation. . . . This means that individual Kpelle are guided by the same expectations in the competition for power. They play by the same rules and for the same stakes, which means that no one goes too far in the means he uses to acquire position. (pp. 229–230)

Perhaps one reason *Malaŋ* is so important in Kpelle culture is its faithful rendition of these twin themes: individual achievement constrained by collective rules.

One of the most frequently heard terms in discussion of people and their actions is usually translated as "sense." The word, however, has at least three meanings to people who use it. The first is "common sense," or the ability to attend and respond to one's environment in the expected way. Children were roughhousing too near a baby and the mother scolded them, "Go away from here, can't you see the baby? You have no sense." A second meaning is intelligence. One informant in discussing *Malaŋ,* said, "You have to have sense to play *Malaŋ.*" Finally, sense refers to wisdom which, in this case would be knowledge of Kpelle custom and ritual. An older person, by virtue of his age, will always have more of this kind of sense than a young person.

Kpelle children's games reflect *and* develop[10] these three kinds of "sense." As we saw in an earlier example, perceived immaturity or lack of seriousness makes it unlikely one will be invited to participate in organized play—especially the more difficult games. Maturity must be complemented by intelligence. As I am sure readers will agree, these games are intel-

[margin note: 3 types of "sense"]

lectually demanding, but there is still ample room for the acquisition, over an extended period, of instrumental knowledge. This knowledge can serve the economic or political needs of one's household, or it can be applied in beating one's opponent in a challenging game of *Malaŋ*. One of the most humbling experiences of my life was to lose repeatedly and quickly (contests between evenly matched players may last hours) to men who were "uneducated" and "illiterate."

The next chapter pursues this issue of uniquely Kpelle values and the way in which certain prominent children's activities function to transmit them.

CHAPTER 7

Dances, Songs, Stories, Proverbs, and the Acquisition of Values

In order to correct their children, parents frequently remind them of
the punishment dealt out to the spider as a result of his tricks.
—HENRIES (1966, p. 1)

My first exposure to dancing was on a farm in the late afternoon. A *kuu* of
approximately 15 women ages 15 to 30 had just spent the day, since sun-
rise, hoeing and planting rice on the *kuu* owner's farm. Their bodies were
covered with dirt and perspiration, and fatigue showed in their faces. Nevertheless, this was the time for dancing. There were two musicians, a
young man playing a medium-sized tom-tom and another man beating
sticks on a 5-gallon tin tied to his waist. They had been playing all day for
the women at work. The women formed a line and began dancing with
slow, swaying movements as they sang. One by one, they broke off from
the line and danced much more vigorously, directly in front of the drum-
mers who would increase the tempo. Women who had worked all day with
infants on their backs did not unload their burdens to dance. They held
their hoes at their sides or out in front of them like staffs, keeping time.
Unfortunately, a downpour interrupted the revelry and everyone ran
home through the pouring rain laughing.

There is a saying to the effect that one cannot have play without *li nee*,
and *li nee* means "joy." It is assumed that young children are always in a
joyful mood or should be and thus their play needs no further antecedent
condition. For teenagers and adults, however, play must be preceded by
some circumstances that have produced a feeling of *li nee*. The dance I
witnessed is a perfect case in point. The women had finished a long hard
and satisfying day's work. The dance that followed is both their reward for

the work and also a visible expression of their joy that the work went well and that it is now over. Had they not danced, this would have been an ominous sign of disenchantment with the *kuu* owner or *kuu* leader. I learned to gauge the mood of the townspeople by the degree and intensity of the moonlight dancing.

In this chapter we examine the role of song, dance, story, and proverb as instructive texts. This is a society in which most rituals are conducted in secret and children, especially, are excluded. We have also seen how rarely parents play the role of teacher. So the moral education of children and, indeed, the informal social control of adults, is dependent on frequent reference to this rich library of texts.

(SINGING AND) DANCING THE NIGHT AWAY

In Gbarngasuakwelle children learn to dance before they can walk. I have seen fathers, especially, hold their infant children under the armpits with their feet lightly resting on their (fathers') knees or on a convenient porch wall and watched as the infants danced to music. The movements of their arms or legs and shoulders were far from random and expressed an explicit, if somewhat clumsy, copy of the movements of the older dancers.

Children spend an increasing amount of their play time dancing, and this peaks at 16 for girls and 11 for boys. Children can be found dancing in the open squares every night that there is bright moonlight (Plate 7.1). Adults are usually spectators to this night dancing, but occasionally they too join. Men and women are more exuberant when they dance and may continue dancing, drinking, and singing long after the children have gone to sleep. My attempts to dance were met with a mixture of amusement and approval, but it served as an entry into close and valuable relationships.

The most common dance form is simply a small circle, usually girls, with a leader who sings the call part of the songs as the rest of the group responds. These groups are composed of 5 to 12 individuals and one or two girls shake *Gbe-kee* (gourd rattles) as they dance. The songs and dance steps are usually improvised and tend to be restrained in girls, less so with boys, and least restrained with adults.

A more formal type of dance which has patterned steps and traditional songs is *Yaloŋ-pilii* (throw little water). *Yaloŋ* is danced by teenagers of both sexes and, less frequently, adults and children ages 8 to 10. The groups are large, numbering perhaps 10 to 20, and because of the size, the

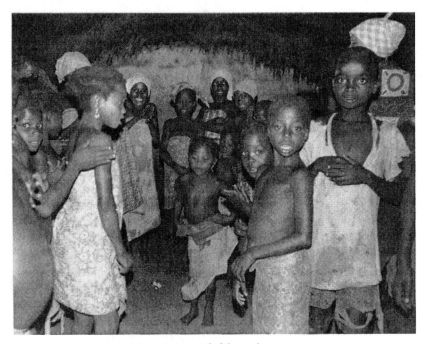

PLATE 7.1. Children dancing.

dance takes place in the mother-ground. Some groups are all male or all female, but generally the sexes are mixed. In fact, several adults told me that the courtship phase of their first marriages began through *Yaloŋ*.

The dancers are arranged in a circle which may remain stationary or move in a counterclockwise direction. One person from the circle runs into the center, does a few "wild" steps, then taps someone else from the circle who repeats the process. The dancers in the circle dance in place raising their feet off the ground in a kind of stamping motion and turn their bodies left and right. They sing a response to a leader's call. Two-line verses are usually repeated over and over. Sometimes children will go around from house to house at dusk gathering dancers for a *Yaloŋ kuu* for the next day, naming the place it will be held. More frequently a couple of dancers gather and sing an advertisement:

Call: "Little-water."
Response: "You all come."

I collected numerous *Yaloŋ* songs, some of which are reproduced below (see also Lancy 1975a). At first, I attempted to record the *Yaloŋ* songs *in situ*, but the chaos and extraneous noise rendered these recordings indecipherable, so I gathered groups of teenage informants to tell me the songs. An interesting sidelight here was that they were virtually incapable of recalling the songs accurately unless they sang them, and some could recall no songs at all unless they were singing and dancing.

Call: "All birds."
Response: "A bird's name [any bird someone can think of] . . . feathers in your hair."

This *Yaloŋ* is similar to the game *Saŋjao, Woni-Kileé* (see Chapter 6). The song continues until the group runs out of bird names, or until the members tire of the song. Some other common *Yaloŋ* verses:

Call: "Oh leopard come let us get down" [from the tree].
Response: "Come let us get down."
Call: "If a person is ugly."
Response: "They put a spoon behind his ear."
Call: "Are we the only ones?"
Response: "*Gba* [a tree] leaves flutter and the ground shakes."

People imitate the movement of the tree and its leaves in the dance.

Call: "Old lover go lie down."
Response: "Count the rafter poles."

There are two variations on the basic *Yaloŋ*: *Loma* (a type of deer) and *Kwala* (monkey). In *Loma*, each dancer hops or leaps through the circle imitating the deer. The verses include:

Call: "*Loma* jumps in the okra patch."
Response: "When you jump you are yourself."
Call: "Hey *Loma*."
Response: "You have given me sense."
Call: "Hey *Loma*."
Response: "They have left me here and gone and I don't have any."
Call: "Frog jumps—baby."
Response: "You don't have a baby and I don't have any."

This expresses the carefree life of the frog and the child who do not have children to care for.

There are numerous "special purpose" songs and dances to accompany the end of bush school, a funeral, the activities of one of the secret societies, and so on. For example, *Jeŋ-kpɛ* is a communal dance associated with the induction phase of initiation. Dancers weave leaves into their hair and garments—representing the bush—as they dance and pass through the town. The call-and-response song tells a tale of love, quarreling, and lust—including graphic descriptions of male and female genitalia—culminating in the birth of the son now being inducted into bush school. Similarly, Richards (1956) reports on the many songs used during the Bemba's *Chisungu* initiation ceremony for young women: "Each woman began to snatch at a *mufungo* bush for leaves . . . [which] they folded into cones to resemble small conical fish traps. They sang a song about setting fish traps and . . . pretended to catch each others finger's in the leaf traps" (p. 65). This is a humorous parable representing fertility. The traps and fingers represent the female and male sexual organs and a song, "The fish has many children and so will the girl" (p. 65), is sung.

Songs do not constitute a separate class of the Kpelle play taxonomy. They are rather encapsulated within the classes of "beating things," "blowing things," and "dances." In fact, there really is no word in Kpelle for song—only for "singing." Songs are always sung in connection with some other activity such as hoeing or dancing and they tend not to have a set beginning and ending. I asked two of my "music informants" to resing songs that I had recorded about 10 days earlier and thus discovered that lyrics were quite variable. Improvisation lent immediacy to the songs as the singers would often include reference to contemporary affairs (literally as well as figuratively) and/or quite personal elements. Gban, for example, built an elaborate song around the conceit of the "mistaken stomach." She fed and cared for a man, bore him a son, but, in the end, he refused to complete their wedding by paying bride-price/service.

Blacking's (1988) reflections on the Venda are typical of views on the function of dance: "The process of increasing participation in dance and music helped Venda children to learn how to think and act, how to feel, and how to relate . . . the underlying principles of the sociocultural system were explained in ways that could be assimilated . . . through communal music and dance" (p. 109). However, I see no such broad instruction of communal principles in Kpelle song. Three more limited ideas seem to be implicated. First, dancing and singing affirm the value of hard work. The Kpelle would not understand our "TGIF," that work is necessary drudgery.[1] Second, a dancing society is a congenial, harmonious society. The Kpelle are quick to shine the social spotlight on sourpusses and cranks.

Third, evening dances provide opportunities for the sexes to safely commingle. There is much teasing and veiled allusion in these encounters, manners are being shaped, and alternative pairings are given a trial and evaluated. Ottenberg (1989), writing about the Nigerian Ibo, describes their dancing songs as "bawdy" and suggests that "the content of the songs may help children to learn sexual rules and constraints" (p. 113).

As always, the little ones cluster on the fringes. Esther Goody (1992), for instance, at a funeral dance in a Ghanaian village, noticed 4-year-old girls swinging and flapping their crooked arms in front of their chest in imitation of older women who flap their pendulous breasts as they dance. In other words, long before the child is old enough to join the dancing circle, he or she attends to and, presumably, learns from both manifest and latent messages embedded in these activities (see also note 1).

STORYTELLING

As often noted in the literature, storytelling has obvious instrumental qualities—there is inevitably a moral. Although not used explicitly as didactic teaching devices or for the recall of oral history, as is the case on Bali (Hobart, 1988), Kpelle folklore clearly serves an enculturative function (Mathews, 1992). Williams (1972/1983), among many others, has written about the close ties between the themes that are prominent in tales and socialization practices. For example, in societies (e.g., Southeast Asia) in which children's aggression is to be restrained, the hero will only display aggression toward outsiders. Kpelle stories touch on the real world, but not for long, as they are inevitably populated by talking animals, "bogeymen," and magicians. Like soap opera, stories never depict harmony or peace, rather there are continual conflicts between man and man, man and woman, and man and nature. However, the variety of genres and the popularity of storytelling suggest that, in Gbarngasuakwelle, it serves recreational and expressive functions as well. An exclusively male pastime among the Kpelle,[2] stories are told mainly on dark or rainy evenings by small groups of men or boys (Plate 7.2).

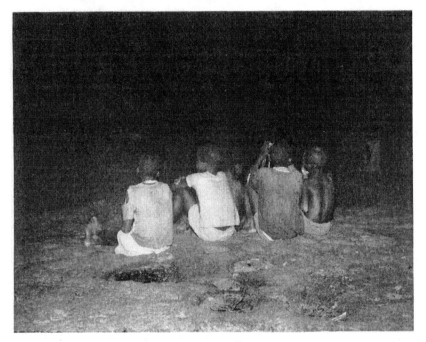

PLATE 7.2. Boys telling stories.

Meni-pele: Folktales with Repeated Elements

The first story form to be described is *Meni-pele*. To distinguish it from other kind of stories, I refer to it as a "folktale." *Meni-pele* is "news play," which is the favorite storyform of young children. *Meni-pele* tales are all relatively simple in content with a limited stock of themes. *Meni-pele* can be quickly identified because they always contain a song. Here is an example from a boy of 13![3]

> Once upon a time there was a man. This man came to a virgin forest. The man said that he was going to cut down the forest to make his farm. They told him he couldn't do this because the forest was enchanted. He said this couldn't be so because he had always set his traps there. The first day he didn't finish cutting the underbrush, but the next morning when he arrived it had all been cut. He was surprised, but began cutting down the trees. He hadn't cut down very many when it grew dark. The next day when he returned he found the trees all cut down. He tried to burn the debris, but the fire kept going out. Again, on his return the next day he found the farm

burned and cleared. He sent his wife to work the ground with her hoe. She did so and by the next day shoots of rice had already appeared. They sent their son to look after the farm. While the boy was there he heard birds singing:

> *Call:* "I made a fine arrow and gave it to Paye's son. Birds don't eat my rice."
>
> *Response:* "*Jau-jau kele ma-jau.*" [The call and response are repeated three times.]

The boy went home and told his father what he had heard, but the father didn't believe him. He beat the boy and put him by the fire. So the man told his wife to go and look after the farm. When she arrived she heard the birds singing: [same song as before]. The woman returned and told her husband what she had heard. He didn't believe her either and, in anger, he beat her and set her beside the fire. The man took a sling and some stones to kill the birds with. He saw the birds in his farm and was preparing to shoot at them when they said, "Wait, hear our song. If it is a bad song, then shoot at us." So the man waited and the birds sang their song: [same song as before]. As the man was listening to the song, his wife came, and seeing him she said, "If you were not a man I would beat you and tie you up and lay you by the fire."

The rice farm or the bush are the most commonly chosen "battle-grounds" for the conflicts and any one of three faults is typically depicted: greed, laziness, and uncooperativeness. This man's greed blinds him to the dangers of making a farm in an enchanted forest and he fails to fully appreciate his helpmates, his son and wife, thus being uncooperative. Ruth Stone (1971/1972), a noted Kpelle folklorist, claims that folktales teach "the young about communal tradition . . ." (p. 32). She recorded a *Meni-pele* about a childless woman who adopts a boy with magical powers. Stone draws out the many lessons about values that are embedded in this particular tale. "In referring to the various animals to be killed the boy says that they are not *hisbaraa-sinaa* or 'male equals.' This term is generally used by a male to refer to a male of the same age and social status" (p. 32).

Telling folktales requires a teller and an audience. *Meni-pele* tellers are almost invariably boys, whereas the audience is composed of other tellers and girls and younger boys. Telling tales complements other types of play. When there is ample light, children engage in "doing play" (*Pele-kee*). With less light (i.e., moonlight) children engage in dancing play such as *Yaloŋ*. When it is dark or raining, children tell tales. A group of four to eight children may gather outdoors on some large rocks at one end of the village, on a porch, on some benches, or indoors to tell tales.

Learning Meni-pele

To find out who knows tales and how they learned them and to build a corpus of tales, nearly every night for 2 weeks, I invited a different group of male and female children of varying ages to my room. Once a group of six to eight children had assembled, I would ask each child, in turn, to tell a story, continuing until quite late in the evening. I recorded the tales and noted the age of the storyteller. I also made notes on the way in which the tales were told. This research allowed me to make several tentative conclusions concerning children's storytelling.

First, girls listen to but do not tell tales. There were always girls present at these recording sessions and they were given ample inducement to tell tales, but none did. Adult informants confirmed this finding and later attempts to solicit tales from adult women also failed. Taking a random sample of 10 girls in the village ages 8 to 13, we asked each girl to tell as many tales as she knew. None would tell us any. An interesting exception to this general trend was the case of a girl of 16 who knew and recounted several tales. This girl, Tono, turned out to be a kind of tomboy. That is, she exhibited many boy-like qualities, including being very argumentative and physically aggressive in fights with boys. She was more than willing to enter into teasing and verbal abuse battles with men, something which girls and even women do only rarely. Many of the villagers spontaneously remarked to me that she would never find a husband because she was too forward. This gender restriction in the access to or display of cultural knowledge is quite common cross-culturally, of course. Gregor (1990) notes that the Mehinaku believe that a girl "cannot learn the basic myths because the words 'will not stay in her stomach'" (p. 484).

Second, among boys, storytelling ability varies considerably, Some boys knew no tales whereas others of the same age knew many. One boy of 10, Moses Weamah, told, in the course of several sessions, 12 different tales. Another boy, Amos Kollie, age 12, also knew many tales. One of his tales follows, with a theme that occurs in many other cultures as well:

> Once upon a time. It concerned a bird. The bird laid its first egg, then the wind came and took the bird away across the ocean. The egg remained in the nest until it hatched. The baby bird managed somehow to feed itself and it lived. When it had grown up it started to look for its mother. This is the song it sang as it was flying:
>
> > *Call:* "The seed, let us go and look for our mother."
> > *Response:* "The seed is up high."

Call: "The wind came and took our mother, let us go and look for our mother."

Response: "The seed is up high."

Call: "The wind came from the south and took our mother. Let us go look for our mother."

Response: "The seed is up high."

The bird met a pigeon. The pigeon cooked dried pigeon for him. After eating it, he told pigeon to try its voice to see whether the pigeon was its mother. The pigeon sang [noises that pigeon makes]. Then he said to her, "You are not my mother," and he flew into the sky again and started to sing [same song as before].

These "units" are then repeated as encounters with the bird with green and red feathers (*Woa*) and hawk (*Kpaaŋ*).

Now he is on the way to his mother. He started his journey with this song: [same song as before]. He came and met his father weaving a mat, but his mother had gone to look for greens for the stew. When she returned, she was very glad to see him. They killed two cows and three goats and had a big feast for him.

This story, like the one in the introduction, is *Meni-pele*. *Meni-pele* have structural features that set them off from the three other story types. They contain a repeated song and the nonsong portion also tends to be a refrain which is modified slightly each time it is repeated. These features make the tales easier to recall. In the first *Meni-pele*, a boy, his mother, and his father listen to birds singing. In Amos's story a little bird meets with various species of birds. This bird-naming theme is also found in the *Saŋjao* game (see Chapter 6) and in one of the *Yaloŋ* songs (see above). In other *Meni-pele* I recorded, the refrain includes various animals trying to climb a palm tree, various animals trying to climb a hill, and a number of men going, one at a time, to fetch water. Finally, *Meni-pele* are told only by boys 12 or younger; older boys tell *Polo-yee* (fables) and *Sia-polo* (riddles).

In addition to this minimally intrusive research, where I merely hosted folk tale evenings, I conducted more in-depth studies (Lancy, 1977a). I was not sure, for example, whether a tale was simply a rough outline or formula which, once learned, could be embellished or modified as the storyteller saw fit? Or, was a tale a relatively fixed entity (or artifact) that would not be altered appreciably from one storyteller to the next, or from one telling to the next? To test these two alternatives I devised a simple experiment.

I had Moses Weamah, a prolific storyteller, tell two folktales which I recorded. Then, 10 days later, I played back the first few lines of each tale for Moses and asked him to tell them to me again. My purpose here was to assess the amount of variation from one telling to the next. There was, in fact, little variation between tellings. A few details were added, a few left out. The second tale involved having various animals try to carry an iron mortar and pestle up a hill. Each tries but only Sali succeeds. The same animals appear in both tellings but the order is changed somewhat, and one more animal is added in the second telling. The implication is that the refrains of the *Meni-pele* are learned as units which can be added on to lengthen a story; such key elements as the names of animals can be changed without altering the character of the story.

In the course of my investigation, I found two other boys (ages 11 and 12) besides Moses who knew quite a few folktales. I conducted in-depth interviews with all three of these boys but found nothing in their backgrounds that set them apart in any way from boys who knew few or no tales. The only thing they shared was an enjoyment of telling and listening to tales—all kinds.

Polo-ɤee Fables: Kpelle "Just So" Stories

Polo-ɤee are either creation stories, or parables with a moral at the end. *Polo-ɤee* are longer and more complex than *Meni-pele* or *Sia-polo*. A boy knows at most two of them, and they are told in gatherings of older children and adults. Although they are more complex and make greater demands on the teller, the message is usually fairly transparent (even I got it), and thus *Polo-ɤee* serve well as moral lessons.

The following is a creation story and was provided by a boy of 11:

> It concerns an old woman. This old woman cooked her rice and said, "The person who will eat this rice will have to carry me to the market." So father spider agreed to eat the rice, then he put the old lady on his back. As they were going along he asked the old lady to get down, but she refused. Then spider said, "Let there be war." The war started and spider said to his attackers, "If you want to throw me down, throw me on my back." They threw him down on his back, cutting his head, but the old woman jumped on his stomach. Spider then said to his attackers, "If you're going to throw me down again, throw me down hard on my stomach." They did this, but the old woman had changed to his back. Then father spider went to the sandcutter [diviner] to find out how he could get the old woman off his back. He

told spider to take her to cut palm nuts. When they got to the palm tree, he told the old woman to get down so he could climb the tree, When she did he ran away and left her there. She died. Spider returned to find only her bones. He took up one of the bones and said, "Here is one of the old woman's bones," whereupon the bone jumped onto the back of his head. So father spider went to the place where the horned birds take their baths. He told the old woman's bone, "Get down so we can take a bath." The bone got off his head and spider ran away. But when the birds came to take a bath, the old woman's bone got on the backs of their heads. Therefore this is how the horned [hornbill] bird got a horn on the back of its head.

A boy of 12 told the following parable, which has a very "mature" and didactic theme[4]:

Once upon a time. It concerns an unfaithful woman. This woman was very unfaithful. Every man she saw she asked him for love. She went and met a fish on the water and asked the fish for love. The fish agreed. She then asked her husband, "What type of soup do you want to eat today?" "Collard greens," he replied. She went back and asked the fish the same question. He told her that he wanted to eat collard greens. She made the greens, but brought the soup to the waterside. Whenever she goes to the waterside she says, "I'm going to draw water." She covers the rice, puts it in a pot, then puts the pot on her head. When she gets there she puts the food down and starts calling the fish. She calls the fish, "*Dom lam lam.*" The fish comes. He eats the rice and she carries the empty pan to town. She continued like this for a long time. Her husband in town asked her to cook a cabbage, She cooked the cabbage and carried it to her "water man" [water spirit]. She mixed dried greens [inferior-tasting food] for her husband in the town. She took the rice to the waterside and started calling the fish, "*Dom lam lam.*" So it came and ate the rice. She took the pot and carried it back in the town. [Her] little child was a twin. He could change himself into anything. So she cooked another rice; while she carried it the child turned himself into a fly and settled on the pot. When they got to the waterside he flew and sat on the leaves and listened to the woman. So the woman put the rice down and started calling the fish which came and ate the food. As the woman carried the empty pot back to town the boy sat on it again. When they got in town, the child went to his father on the farm and told all about the woman. The woman who always cooked the rice and carried it to the waterside was going on *kuu*. So the husband dressed himself like a woman, put on all the things a woman wears, took his gun and put it at his side. He cooked and took food to the waterside. He started calling the fish. The fish thought it was his girl-friend, and he came. He was about to eat the rice, when the man stepped back and shot him, The man took it into town and cooked it. He kept some

for the woman, when she came he gave it to her. The woman took this food
to the waterside; she didn't know that he had killed her boy friend. When she
got to the waterside she started calling her boyfriend. Each time she called
the water rose higher and she kept calling until the water covered her head.
So it is with a woman who does not stay with one man,

Telling *Polo-yee* involves the use of a wide variety of dramatic gestures
and frequent change of tone for emphasis. When the boy was telling the
spider story he slapped his hands on the ground and said "Crack" to accompany the spider's being thrown down. The boy telling the unfaithful
woman story stood up and cupped his hands around his mouth as he
called, "*Dom lam lam.*" When he described the boy's turning into a fly his
voice dropped to a conspiratorial whisper.

Although most boys did not know very many *Polo-yee,* I wanted to see
whether they held the appropriate story schema in memory. My assistant
and I made up a novel *Polo-yee*—the "Duck Story"—that was faithful to
the model. He read it to a group of 20 boys every Sunday and asked them
(individually) to recall it every Friday for 3 weeks. We found evidence that
the boys held a *Polo-yee* schema in memory: "Even when recall was very
poor (only 10% of the best performance) the theme was intact and original elements were used in the appropriate places. . . . Hence, with each
new trial, [boys] told a longer story which was also a more complete copy
of the original" (Lancy, 1977a, p. 302).

Sia-polo: Riddles and Argument

The Kpelle are continually litigious and greatly value erudition and cleverness in public debate (see Chapter 4). They love to tell riddles or *Sia-polo.*
Roberts and Forman (1971) define the riddle as a "puzzling question" presented by one person to another, often as a game: "participation in riddling . . . about how to handle oneself under interrogation and how to in-
terrogate others" (p. 529). *Sia-polo* set up several competing choices for
resolution. At the end, a question is asked of the listeners, such as, "Of
these three men who should get the girl?", which the participants must resolve through argument. The following were told by boys of 10 and 11:

> STORYTELLER: Once upon a time. It concerns two men. These men had a lot
> of fleas on them. One said, "I have more fleas than you," to the other
> man. Then he took a pan and held it under his arm and the fleas filled
> it up. Then the second man took his trousers off and the fleas just car-

ried them away to the garbage dump. If this so which of these two men had more fleas?

GROUP: Both have an equal amount of fleas.

STORYTELLER: I agree.

STORYTELLER: It concerns three men. These three men had an argument about stealing. One said to the others, "I can steal better than you." The other two said, "No, you can't steal more than us." They went and found a dove sitting on its eggs. One man climbed the tree and stole the eggs, unknowing to the dove. He put the eggs in his mouth. While climbing down, his friend stole the eggs from his mouth The friend carried the eggs in his hand, but as he was climbing down the third man stole the eggs from his hand. If this is so, of these three men who can steal the best?

BOY OF 12: The person who stole the eggs from the other's mouth, he is the one that can steal the best

GROUP: They all can steal.

STORYTELLER: They all can steal.

As *Meni-pele* is the preferred story of young children, so *Sia-polo* is the preferred form of men. Not every man knows *Polo-yee* and very few can do *Wei-meni-pele* (epics), but every boy learns a few *Sia-polo*. More important, one does not need to know *Sia-polo* to participate in the argument that follows the story.

I invited four men and two women ages 28 to 35 and a young man of 17 to tell riddles one night. Fueled with plenty of palm wine, the riddlers held a session that lasted nearly 4 hours. This is the first story that was told:

AKEWOLI-LA (male): There were three young men who approached a girl for love. The girl agreed. After the girl agreed, they left and went down to the city to work. Payday came, so when they went to the paymaster, one told the white man, "The work I did for you, pay me with a mirror." One said to him, "Give me powder," and the other man said, "Pay me with one of the sheepskins you have." So the man took those three things and gave it to the three of them. So they went into the town. The man who had the mirror looked in it and found that their lover had died. They said, "What can we do?" The man with the sheepskin said, "Come let's sit on the sheepskin." As soon as they sat on it they arrived at the place. They were about to lower the body into the grave. The man with the powder sprinkled it on the woman and she got up and sat down. Therefore, I'm asking my friends, of these three men who is the woman for?

KPO-KPALA (male): As for me, my opinion, the man who had the sheepskin, the woman belongs to him.

AKEWOLI-LA: How about the powder owner?

KPO-KPALA: The person who had the powder is just a medicine man for that woman.

AKEWOLI-LA: The person who saw the dead body?

KPO-KPALA: Does it mean that when someone sees a dead body, they bring it to life? When someone sees a dead body, then he has not brought that person back to life.

YAKPAWLO (male): Those three men you talk about, the woman is wife to all of them. "If a person hasn't made a rice farm, he can't cut the rice." This is the answer, The man who looked in the mirror and saw the dead body. They went there. Their friend put the powder on her and she got up and sat down.

KPO-KPALA: I ask him why. You said the woman is for the three of them. He said, "The man who saw the dead body and the man whose sheepskin they sat on and the man who put the powder on her." So I asked him, "If someone sees a dead body, does that mean he has brought the person back to life?"

AKEWOLI-LA: The woman belongs to those three men.

KPO-KPALA: I can't agree to that. What I agree to is that the person who put the skin down and all sat on it.

AKEWOLI-LA: If they had come home and they had already buried the woman, and the powder had not been there, you think that if someone brings a sheepskin he has brought that person back to life? How about the person that saw the dead body?

KPO-KPALA: If someone sees a dead body with his eyes does it mean he has brought the person back to life?

AKEWOLI-LA: Can you see someone die if you are in Firestone [rubber plantation]?

KPO-KPALA: I can't see a dead body from Firestone.

AKEWOLI-LA: She is for three of them.

KPO-KPALA: If there are three men on one woman where can they take her?

AKEWOLI-LA: Only God can take her from them.

This *Sia-polo* is a fairly standardized one that I collected with little variation from several storytellers. It differs here in that Akewoli-la has added his own beginning to it. Generally, it starts out simply: One man had a mirror, a second had a sheepskin, and so on. Akewoli-la has added an original and a clearly foreign (i.e., non-Kpelle) introduction. The argument following the *Sia-polo* was quite long and rather lively. Not all riddles had this open-ended quality. One that I collected—which shows up in other folklore collections—asks how a man can ferry a leopard, a goat, and cassava across the river taking only two of them at a time. Interestingly, boys seem more willing to jump in during the argument when these more puzzle-like *Sia-polo* are offered.

Learning to Riddle

Riddles are short and easy to remember, but extracting the rule or moral is difficult to articulate—just the opposite of fables or *Polo-yee*. Further, boys seem to begin their acquisition of *Sia-polo* in adolescence—much like *Malaŋ*. The first two *Sia-polo* were recorded during two structured sessions of riddle telling with 20 boys drawn randomly from the population of 9- to 13-year-olds in the town. They were divided into two groups of 10, which met on consecutive nights. My research assistant and I explained to each group that they were to tell *Sia-polo* and that we would give them 2 cents for each story. Using random orders, each boy was called on to tell a riddle if he knew any. After the riddles, time was allowed for argument. After each boy had a chance, they were called on again randomly until all boys had exhausted their store. The total number of riddles generated in the two evenings was 22. None of the 9-year-olds could supply any and among the 10 to 13-year-olds, the range was from 0 to 3 with a mean of 1.4 riddles.

After age 9, there was no association between age and number of riddles told. Not all the riddles were equally "good." A few were not *Sia-polo* at all but seem to have been made up on the spot under the pressure of competition and the 2 cents reward. Some were incomplete. Furthermore, unlike their adult counterparts, the boys did not spend a great deal of time "arguing." The group generally tended to agree that "all were equal" at the end of each *Sia-polo*. Others who have observed children telling and/or listening to riddles see them as making an important contribution to enculturation. "Dusun children also learn and often use a great many riddles as part of their play . . . [these] serve the functions of channeling social conflicts, reducing interpersonal aggression, teaching rules of social action, validating the Dusun system of culture, explaining the world . . ." (Williams, 1969, p. 85).

Margaret Read (1960) noted how important erudition is to the Ngoni—Bantu-speaking cattle herders from central Africa—and, not surprising, riddles are an important element of children's folklore. Children of both sexes, but separately, told riddles in the evening: "They jeered at slow or inept relies, and applauded correct answers. An unexpected reply . . . often drew applause, even if it was not the accepted correct answer . . . It was clear that riddles were . . . a test of intelligence and of memory . . ." (pp. 97–98).

Riddling is also related to "the art of speaking . . . regarded as a basic Ngoni characteristic" (Read, 1960, p. 146).

The dilemmas presented in the riddle parallel, in structure, the dilemmas that occur daily in the household and town—over rights, responsibilities and relationships. Anywhere two or more people gather discussion revolves around some simmering issue—issues that often end up in court. Talking matter (Chapter 4) or court proceedings are a common occurrence and provide opportunities for the Kpelle to display their eloquence and rhetorical ability (Lancy, 1980c). These texts resemble closely the kinds of arguments brought forth in *Sia-polo*.

Wei-meni-pele: The Epitome of Kpelle Oral Literature

Wei-meni-pele roughly translates as "unending news play." A single storyteller will entertain a crowd of people for hours, often all night, with *Wei-meni-pele*. The key feature of this storyform is the description of the various animals and their traits. There are two aspects to every animal: its "natural history" or its normal behavior pattern within some natural setting, which includes its habits and signaling devices (such as bird songs), and its "supernatural history," which includes the traits and behaviors ascribed to it by humans (such as a leopard's stupidity and Sali's cleverness). The storyteller has to be well versed in both the natural and supernatural history of animals. He also sings songs interspersed with the stories. He makes lewd jokes, and, finally, he must be able to weave his audience and their personalities, foibles, and physical characteristics into the narrative.

Kerkula, a *Ƶò*, was a noted storyteller, I recorded several hours of his Wei-meni-pele to an audience composed mostly of young people. He seemed to be playing a mock-serious role of "educator" to these young people. As he talked he continually admonished them to listen carefully or would call on one of them to pay particular attention and then say, "Now isn't that so?" The audience responded enthusiastically to him and to his stories and at least half the time they were laughing *at* him. He was more than a little inebriated and seemed consciously playing the role of "clown." Excerpts from Kerkula's *Wei-meni-pele* can be found in Lancy (1975a). Ruth Stone (1988) also recorded what she refers to as *Woi-meni-pele*, or epic storytelling, and describes the life of Kulung, a master of the genre, who had himself been apprenticed to a *Woi* master. Stone makes the interesting observation that while the young produce song, dance, and story; the old contribute as well by serving as critics. It is the "elders who comprehend the subtleties of the performance and the layered references" (p. 95).

I estimate that the typical Kpelle hears two to three dozen of these moralizing folktales, each on numerous occasions over the course of childhood. They also listen to adults debating *Sia-polo* (riddles) on many occasions and, more rarely, will sit enthralled listening to a master of the epic story form. Further and fairly extensive research (Lancy, 1977a) indicated that boys gradually improve their own ability to tell folktales and parables and acquire a repertoire of stories to tell over the period from ages 9 to 15. Altogether, folklore provides an extensive and thorough education in Kpelle values.[5]

PROVERBS

It is early evening on our verandah and Chief Wollokollie is relating the day's *Koti-meni-saa*, or court business. In addition to the several adult listeners, there are the inevitable toddlers and young children—at the breast, between the knees, underfoot. One 4-year-old is a little fussy and refuses to sit still and his mother admonishes him, "Sit quietly to learn the crocodile's tricks."

Proverbs "are concerned with morality, with evaluating and shaping courses of action . . ." (White, 1987, p. 151). As such, they are widely employed in teaching children the rules of the society as well as how to become accepted within society. The Chaga (Raum, 1940), for example, believe that proverbs are only effective teaching "aids" after the child has reached the age of about 14. Prior to that age, folktales are the preferred medium. The Kpelle are extremely liberal in the didactic use of proverbs, much like the Ngoni:

> In a mixed gathering of children and adults, a proverb might suddenly be dropped like a stone into a pond. The conversation rippled away into silence,

and the boy or girl who had refused to share some peanuts or had been boasting began to wonder to himself: "Can that be for me? No? Yes? It is me. I am ashamed." No one said anything but the shamed one took the first chance of slipping away to avoid further public notice. The use of proverbs in this way were an effective way of making a child learn for himself and apply the lesson; and with children, as with adults, the use of proverbs was a way of "saving face" when a direct rebuke in the presence of others would have caused overwhelming shame. (Read, 1960, pp. 44–45)

The Kpelle also take care that children learn proverbs (*Saŋ*) as well as the lessons the proverbs teach. However, Kulah (1973), who studied proverb learning among Kpelle youth, claims, "We never obtained any reports of a session purposely designed to teach children proverbs or how they are applied" (p. 91). This is done via *Koloŋ*, a "miscellaneous" play-form under "doing play." It is a game in which two teams challenge each other to provide the appropriate paired-response phrase to an offered stimulus phrase. *Koloŋ* represents an interesting and apparently unique type of folklore. It is essentially a verbal memory game. Like some stories and songs, doing *Koloŋ* requires the learning of and production of linked phrases. At the same time, because it is a game played by two teams with a winning and a losing side, it incorporates some elements of strategy.

Teams are composed of one to eight players of both sexes who vary in age from 8 years and up. Adults do not play, but they may critique play from the sidelines and supply fresh *Koloŋ*, as needed (Kulah, 1973). There are two parts to the *Koloŋ*. The first part, a stimulus phrase, is called *Koloŋ*. The second part, a response phrase, is called answer but is actually a proverb (*Saŋ*). One team starts by having one of its members tell a *Koloŋ*, or stimulus part. The other team members confer and try to supply the correct answer or response part to match the offered *Koloŋ*. If they succeed, they gain a point and they now offer a *Koloŋ*. If they fail, the first team must give the correct response and they gain a point and get to offer the next *Koloŋ*. The initiative shifts only when one team successfully matches the other team's *Koloŋ*. The game is played at night and may continue for ½ to 2 hours. The more players per team, the higher the number of pooled *Koloŋ* and the longer play can continue. (For a more detailed description of how the game is played, see Kulah, 1973, pp. 97–99.)

As with so much of play, especially that of children, the extraneous noise and commotion made it difficult to record and interpret *Koloŋ* while a game was in progress. Therefore I resorted to a more structured approach to gathering and studying them. Four individuals were selected randomly from each of the following populations: girls 8 to 10 years old, boys 8 to 10 years old, girls 11 to 13 years old, boys 11 to 13 years old. Four individuals were also selected from the following populations: girls 14 to 20 years old, boys 14 to 20 years old, women 30 years +, and men 30 years +, for a total of 32 individuals. Each person was interviewed individually and asked to tell as many *Koloŋ* as he or she knew and they were paid 5 cents for each one. Specifically, we collected (1) *Koloŋ*, (2) answers, and (3) explanations for the answers. The explanations were sought because I knew that the answers were proverbs and I was anxious to learn whether individual comprehension of proverbs would vary with age or sex.

A total of 87 distinct *Koloŋ* pairs were collected. Individuals produced from a minimum of three to a maximum of 20. The average for the 32 informants was 7.66. Four examples are shown below:

#1 K: I cut the cassava and the inside was white.
    A: Snails don't have bones.
#2 K: I fall this way and I fall that way.
    A: A calabash can't say it won't sit under the palm wine.
#3 K: A spark flies out from the fire.
    A: A pepper is small but its burn is strong.
#4 K: Under the water is a short drum.
    A: A short man can't measure himself in deep water.

Males ($n = 16$) produced significantly more *Koloŋ* pairs than females ($n = 16$) 10.31 versus 5.5. Young informants (8 to 13 years old, $n = 16$) produced fewer *Koloŋ* pairs than older informants (14+ years old, $n = 16$): 6.9 versus 8.9. As with other types of play, females are less involved than males, Females do not play *Koloŋ* as often as males; therefore they knew fewer of them. Older people play *Koloŋ* rarely but know more of them because of their apparent accumulation in memory over time.

Some *Koloŋ* pairs were offered by only a single informant, whereas others were given by as many as 20 informants. The average number of times a *Koloŋ* pair was offered among the 32 informants was three. Where the same pair was recorded from several individuals, they tended to be exactly alike, indicating that the phraseology of *Koloŋ* and the answer, as well as the pairing, are very stable.

A rather extensive content analysis (Lancy, 1975a) revealed no association between themes in the stimulus and response parts. This would suggest that the *Koloŋ* must be learned as pairs; that there are no clues in the stimulus part that would allow one to guess at or construct the response part.

Explanations given by informants to the response or proverb parts of the *Koloŋ* fell into three categories. The first category was simply, "I don't know," as an answer. The second category consisted of explanations that derived from the context depicted in the response itself (EC). The third category of explanations was abstract or normative (EN). These EN explanations were in keeping with the "use" to which proverbs are put, namely, when norms are invoked. Three *Koloŋ* pairs follow and indicate typical "contextual" and "normative" explanations

K: I pass this way and I pass that way.
A: There is a path in every quarter.
EC: The town is cleared all over and there isn't any underbrush.
EN: Every man has his superior, so that if a man beats a small boy, someone will be there to beat him, too.

K: There is a young banana at the waterside.
A: A young girl is known by her breasts.
EC: Before a girl comes to womanhood, her breasts must come up.
EN: People are known for what they can do.

K: Behind our house is good palm-leaf fabric.
A: Women's necks are used to carrying heavy loads.
EC: Because their necks are thick.
EN: What you practice at is hard for you to forget.

Eight- to 13-year-old children give, "I don't know" (63%) and contextual answers (37%). Fourteen- to 20-year-olds are transitional. They realize that an explanation is called for; hence, they almost never say, "I don't know," but only 40% of their explanations are normative. The percentage of normative explanations for adults increases to 60%. Actually, the adults were all under 40; it is quite possible that with an older group the normative proportion would have been even higher. What seems to be happening then is that children first learn the response parts of *Koloŋ* simply as the answer part of the pair. Later they begin to understand that these answer parts may be used in other contexts and have "meaning." By age 14 they have learned that the answer parts are also proverbs. They also have learned that proverbs embody "rules" which can be extracted from them. The same proverb may supply different "rules" depending on when and where it is used; what is important in learning to understand proverbs is that they almost always must be "interpreted" or explained.

SUMMARY AND CONCLUSIONS

Songs, stories, and *Koloŋ* are all parts of the Kpelle expressive culture. Of the four story types in use, folktales are told by young boys; riddles are told by older boys and men, although only men fully "argue" them; and fables and epic tales are told by a few older boys and men and require special skills to execute properly. As with other aspects of the culture (e.g., work skills), some stories are widely shared and others are not. *Meni-pele* tales appear to be stored in the minds of nearly all young boys and *Sia-polo* riddles are stored in the minds of nearly all older boys and men. Not all these individuals have the capacity, however, to retrieve stories on demand. *Polo-yee* fables and *Wei-meni-pele* epic tales, on the other hand, require not only an extensive knowledge of various story contents, but also several skills that must be applied to achieve their proper execution. This knowledge and skill combination is stored in the minds of only a few of the males in Gbarngasuakwelle. Interestingly, my investigation revealed that the males who have stored and can retrieve on demand *Polo-yee* and *Wei-meni-pele* are also likely to possess such other esoteric or rare information as in medicine making, rituals, and certain songs.

Three types of songs were discerned: short, fixed songs, which are the most frequently heard especially in connection with dancing and rituals; long, totally improvised songs, sung by people when they are alone or by young girls in groups; and, long, partially improvised songs, sung by a few accomplished singers.

Some adults are notable singers and are often sought out for their singing ability. I studied two such singers, a male and a female. Their virtuosity appears to lie less in voice quality or memory for song content than in the ability to maintain rhythm and carefully improvise as they sing.

In *Koloŋ* we have a fascinating display of "indirect" learning. Children acquire *Koloŋ* pairs in the course of playing the game. The number of *Koloŋ* known gradually increases with age, with men knowing more *Koloŋ* than women. What is more interesting is that young children do not understand that the response parts of the *Koloŋ* are proverbs; adolescents fully appreciate this fact and virtually all attempt to explain their meaning; but only the older subjects have a full appreciation of the meaning and use of proverbs. These findings are completely consistent with those of Kulah's (1973) study of the acquisition and use of proverbs among the Kpelle. He speaks of proverbs as "pedagogic and judicial . . . tools" (p. 12). As important as proverbs are to the Kpelle, Kulah "never obtained any reports of a session purposely designed to teach children proverbs or how they are applied" (p. 91). Instead, the *Koloŋ* game provides the child with a "vast store" of proverbs, which he or she will gradually learn to use in context.

Although it is fairly easy to discern Kpelle values embedded in their folklore, I was most forcibly struck by the connection to "talking matter" (Chapter 4, this volume; Lancy, 1980c). When young boys tell *Meni-pele* tales, they are frequently challenged by the other boys with such expressions as "What do you mean?" or "How do you know, were you there?" or "That's not possible." These comments are made in jest, but the teller will pause in his or her narrative to answer them. The challenge for the teller lies in being able to return to the tale and to continue narrating smoothly from the point where he or she left off. This is not easy. In the court there are four occasions when a participant may engage in a lengthy narrative; what I have labeled the "self-evident," "staged-anger," "penitent," and "expository" speech events (Lancy, 1980c). All these speech events have expressive functions; that is, they are designed to sway the audience in the speaker's favor. Frequently, however, during one of the speeches, the speaker will be interrupted by another participant who asks a pointed question—"What are you saying?" "When did this happen?"—or makes a joke at the speaker's expense. If these outbursts are not successfully fielded by the speaker and if the speaker cannot easily resume his or her speech, the impact the speaker was trying to achieve is lost. A requirement common to both *Meni-pele* and talking matter is verbal agility in the face of a hostile audience.

With *Polo-ɤee*, or fables, more parallels between telling stories and talking matter emerge. In *Polo-ɤee*, one must hold an audience's attention for some time (i.e., they are long). This is primarily accomplished by dramatizing the events depicted. Gestures, changes in speech tone, even facial expressions are part of the performance. Because the content of the stories is generally familiar to the audience, their attention may wander if the teller is unskilled. Much the same process occurs in the court. When a participant gives a self-evident, staged anger, or penitent speech, the longer he or she can hold the court's attention the better the outcome will be. As in *Polo-ɤee*, the audience already knows the "story," but they will listen and not interrupt if the speaker is sufficiently dramatic in making his or her speech.

Sia-polo riddles would seem to be the perfect play model for talking matter, The stories themselves are usually familiar. As in a trial, the "evidence" is quickly presented and then may not be referred to again. What preoccupies the participants is the argument that ensues. As in a trial, sides are quickly taken. If the story presents a conflict between two men, then, in the argument, one person will "defend" one of these men and another participant will "defend" the other, each providing a rationale for his protagonist's position. Storytelling, then, may very well serve as a training ground for talking matter. A significant fact is that women who participate only rarely in the courts are also only occasionally involved in storytelling.

The "elders" in a dispute add two substantial speech elements to the contest, jokes and proverbs. These jokes and proverbs are designed to wound the speaker, to lower his or her esteem in the eyes of the audience. The use of joking is begun early by young boys, and at times it is difficult to distinguish between joking and abusing, A boy may make a joke about another boy, "He walks like a goat," which evokes laughter from other boys in the group. The boy thus attacked is angry and may respond with, "Your father's big penis," which is an expression of abuse. There are, in other words, no jokes told that do not have an obvious "victim." Proverbs are not used as such by children. In playing *Koloŋ*, however, they do acquire a substantial store of proverbs, which they may later use in talking matter. Proverbs and, to a lesser extent, jokes involve both language and ideology. That is, both are structured speech events, and both can take on extended meaning (i.e., ideology) when used in disputes. Children learn the syntax of proverbs and jokes in their play, but learning the semantics or meanings of jokes and proverbs comes only through exposure to and participation in adult play and talking matter.

Up to this point, I have described cultural routines that function indirectly in preparing children for adulthood. These are stories of play. In the next chapter we turn to situations in which children learn to do adult work by doing child work. That is, the Kpelle, like most societies that use some means other than schooling to enculturate, have an exquisitely detailed program of chores for children that are graded by age and gender. Chapter 8, considers the chore curriculum.

CHAPTER 8

Children's Work

If one asks a Chaga where he got his knowledge, in nine cases out of ten, the reply is: "From nobody; I taught myself!"

—RAUM (1940, pp. 246–247)

Every small [Tallensi] boy of 6–7 years and upwards has a passionate desire to own a hen.

—FORTES (1970, p. 20)

No one teaches a girl to wield a hoe. Her first observation of hoeing occurs when she is still wrapped on her mother's back in a lappa. The rhythmic movements no doubt rock her to sleep. Before she can walk, she will repeatedly grasp a stick while she is sitting on the ground and lift it up and then bring it down on the ground ("practice play"; Piaget, 1951) in a manner clearly imitative of her mother and the other women she's watching. She may get her first real hoe at age 6. The first time she uses a hoe she will have little difficulty in using it, and, from then on, when her mother is hoeing, she'll be hoeing. The same is true for the boy and his machete.

No one teaches a young girl how to carry water. She will toddle after her older sisters to the stream and, as soon as she is stable enough on her legs, someone will place a small pan on her head and fill it with water and she will carry it home. She has seen it done and, with practice and increasing strength and stature, the pan she can carry will grow larger. Likewise for boys carrying firewood on their heads. The young child carries out simple tasks that he or she has seen performed on a daily basis since birth. There is no teaching and proficiency depends entirely on maturation and practice. As White's (1959) theory suggests, children, evidently, find the opportunity to imitate and serve their elders intrinsically rewarding. Family members encourage this tendency by helping children manage scaled-down versions of common chores. In short, we see much the same picture, set against the backdrop of the mother-ground, we examined in children's aquisition of various playforms.

On the other hand, when such intrinsic motivation is apparently lacking, parents and older siblings display limited tolerance and are quick to employ chastisement in some form. This may range from a mild rebuke, perhaps couched as a proverb (see Chapter 7, note 1), to a severe beating. Consistent with what one sees in other agrarian societies, Kpelle children are viewed as economic assets. Bledsoe (1980) notes: "Kpelle women . . view their children . . as resources rather than impediments . . whose labor will lighten their burdens and offer them security in their old age" (p. 3); "the labor of children increases the productivity of their parent's farms" (p. 59); "children are a form of property that fathers must pay for and maintain if they are to be considered legal owners" (p. 91).

As we shall see, some forms of work or skills, such as hammock making, are *optional*. The child will not be chided for failing to practice his hammock making. On the contrary, if a boy wants to learn this skill he may have a hard time finding a willing tutor. However, the work of the household is mandatory.[1] Viewing culture as information (Chapter 2), we can see that the Kpelle expect that certain kinds of information or skills will be mastered by everyone (of the appropriate gender); other skills are open to those with the initiative to pursue them; and access to yet other information/skill is restricted (e.g., bush school and apprenticeship).

A DEVELOPMENTAL PERSPECTIVE ON CHILDREN'S WORK

Children from the age of 4 are expected to begin to make a contribution to the economic life of the household. Perhaps the most common speech event employed by adults with 4- to 5-year-olds is the order to "fetch and carry." Boys and girls are given small woven bags or carryalls to use for their own things as well as to transport small amounts of food from one household to another or from the town to the farm. Or, they are sent to buy or sell items (discussed later). As meals are being prepared and consumed there is a great deal of shuttling back and forth as food is moved from preparation area to cooking fire to diners—who may be scattered about the compound or seated haphazardly on logs littering a farm site. Young children are the primary servers.

From age 5 on, boys are expected to fetch and carry firewood and may be given one-third size machetes (cutlass in Liberian English) to reduce overly long branches to carryable length. Girls from that age fetch water in pans or gourds and begin to hull rice in a small mortar and pestle.

At age 6, boys and girls are entrusted with the primary care of their 2- to 4-year-old siblings. Also at this age, girls will care for infants while they are sleeping, freeing their mother to do such active, heavy work as weeding. Girls are expected to join older siblings in periodic "sweeps" of the house and surrounding territory. Boys pitch in to assist with building construction and maintenance. On the farm, girls weed around the rice, pile up waste to be burned, and carry rice stalk bundles to the storage "kitchen." Boys help with brush cutting and fence building prior to planting and are primarily responsible for pest control—especially chasing away birds—as the crop ripens.

Of course, they are still allowed to be children. Boys, especially, are permitted to play while others around them are working, as long as their play does not interfere with the work and as long as they help when asked. Also, children who are hurt while working will be comforted or, perhaps, teased to stop their crying and toughen them.

However, as Howard (1970) notes for a South Pacific group, "Rotumans seem to be optimists regarding childhood accidents, do not share [our] attitude of caution . . . it is common to see a 3–4 yr. old . . . swinging a razor sharp machete in imitation of his elders" (p. 33). Anthropologists have often observed, with thinly disguised anguish, the seeming lack of concern for children's safety on the part of village people. The resolution of this paradox lies in the society's great reliance on the child's inherent motivation to imitate adults. People have so little time and energy to "waste" on being teachers to the young that they have to rely on the child's curiosity and desire for mastery to propel it forward toward competent practice. This is in contrast to mainstream U.S. society, where parents are the primary teachers and act to restrict children's access to objects/places that may be harmful or inappropriate (Valsiner, 1984).[2]

One of the first things one notices about children learning to work are the opportunities for children to become "peripherally" involved (cf. Lave & Wenger, 1991). Take trapping as an example. At first, the boy merely tags along, as his father checks his traps, learning to attend to the salient stimuli of game and bush (for a parallel case, see Ocitti, 1973, pp. 85–86). Later, he will help his father gather materials to make the trap, then he assists in making and setting them. All this while, there is little verbal interchange between the two. The father expects the boy to learn by observing. Then, the son will try to make his own trap. He can expect to get some advice and criticism from his father but not much. Unlike in U.S. society, the father is not held "responsible" for his son becoming a good trapper as much as he is expected, out of a sense of filiation, to offer the son some assistance. But, the boy's success at becoming a trapper is entirely in his own hands.

At age 7 (see Table 8.1) a boy may be able to construct a simple trap for catching small birds (*Faaŋ*). Each year thereafter, he will probably take on one or two new traps until he has mastered the whole arsenal of 15+ traps. At age 14 he may join *Gbliŋ Gbe*, the boys' hunting society, and learn secret medicines to use in his traps. At age 16 he traps by himself and contributes part of his catch to the family larder.[3]

Enculturation is, for the most part, public. For example, whatever stage our aspiring trapper is at, he will have ample opportunity to observe the efforts of those at more advanced stages—a model of the next level of proficiency is usually available. This was especially evident in the acquisition of weaving (discussed later). Another evident example is mothering. Riesman (1992) observes in another West African society:

> All women caring for their first babies will have had years of experience taking care of babies already under the watchful and sometimes severe eyes of their mothers, aunts, cousins or older sisters. The other women around them will immediately notice, comment on, and perhaps strongly criticize any departure from customary behavior on the part of mothers . . . *deviations hardly have any chance to develop so long as most of the work of child care takes place in the public arena.* (p. 111, emphasis added)[4]

Work is "staged" in another sense and these unspoken customs subtly guide developing individuals in making intelligent choices in terms of where they invest their time and energy. As we have seen, small children carry water and firewood and make market. Older children cook, care for infants, and trap small animals. Young to middle-age individuals work on *kuus*, cut palm nuts, weave nets, and build kitchens. Old people weave fish traps, talk matter, and make medicines.

The stages associated with advancing age are not clearly marked, but one can discern certain broad characteristics associated with each stage. Young children are expected to follow orders. Older children may take some initiative but have no real responsibility. Young men and women are expected to manage their own affairs, but they make few major decisions including whom they will marry. Middle-age men and women delegate work to younger family members and manage household affairs. Old men and women no longer do much work or make day-to-day decisions, but they are expected to be wise and to dispense their sought-after counsel to those younger than themselves. In short, there is no virtue in precocity.

THE TRANSITION FROM PLAY TO WORK

In many societies there is a gradual and subtle transition as children take on more and more responsibility. In Chapter 5, we observed children playing at adult work. In this example, from the Tallensi (a Ghanian people), boys begin to contribute their small share to subsistence, but they do so in a manner that suggests that they are playing, not working:

> When a small boy goes out hunting for fieldmice or birds, if he happens to have a "shrine" he will "give it water," i.e. pour a libation to it. Ashes represent flour, which is stirred up in water as in a real sacrifice. He invokes the shrine, "My father . . . accept this water and grant that I have successful hunting. If I kill an animal, I will give you a dog." Some time later he may catch a live mouse, and when he has played with it to satiety he "sacrifices" it on his shrine—this is the promised "dog." (Fortes, 1970, p. 68)

Harkness and Super (1986) studied the Kipsigis, an East African Nilotic group, and observed: "A game of tag could take place in the context of watching the cows . . . a child might climb a tree while looking after a younger sibling" (p. 99). They found that, from age 2 years to 8 years, the percentage of time children spent in play decreased from 40% to 10%, while work increased from 12% to 50%.

Several researchers have examined the play–work continuum as a function of gender (Edwards & Whiting, 1980). For example, Bloch and Adlers (1994) found, in a Senegalese village, that girls were more likely than boys to engage in "play work," girls transitioned from play to work earlier than boys, and girls were more likely than boys to be called away from play to work. This distinction seems to hold up in many societies (Whiting & Edwards, 1988) and it certainly applies in Kpelle society.

The literature also includes societies in which the subsistence base is quite thin and children are expected to make a substantial contribution at an early age. Among the Yucatec Maya in the Chiapas Highlands, where population exceeds carrying capacity, "the opportunity for play of any sort is relatively limited . . . children as young as three or four are often given chores . . . by age six or seven they are kept busy with work for long periods of time" (Gaskins & Göncü, 1992, p. 31). Friedl (1992) describes the almost continuous drudgery experienced by a 9-year-old Kurdish girl who must steal 10 minutes from her round of clothes washing, water carrying, child minding, cooking, and goat milking to play a game of jacks. The Hadza, a Tanzanian hunting and gathering people, expect children as young as 3 to begin foraging independent of their mothers. By age 5, they gather about half their own caloric needs; by 10 they are completely self-sufficient (Blurton-Jones, 1993). Adults are largely intolerant of children's play.

In general, it appears that "women whose work load goes beyond housework and childcare expect more help from their children. . . . This is true even in American families, as found in many studies of employed mothers" (Whiting & Edwards, 1988, p. 97). In Gbarngasuakwelle, there is considerable intervillage variation. The larger the household and the wealthier the head of household, the more hands there are and the greater the surplus. A woman with co-wives, whose husband's largesse permits the boarding of other unmarried men and women, carries a lighter load and her children will, consequently, have greater freedom from work as well. This freedom from household work not only translates into more time for play; it also affords children the luxury of acquiring such valued but optional skills as weaving. In the next two sections, I explicate the chore curriculum by examining how children learn weaving and marketing.

LEARNING TO WEAVE

Weaving in Gbarngasuakwelle is a wonderful venue for the observation of enculturation. There are a great variety of woven products in the society and these vary in complexity and in the gender of the weaver. Nyenpu is 8 years old and she is trying to learn to weave a fishnet. Her mother, Yau-Sua, is her teacher. (Plate 8.1). Nyenpu first expressed an interest in net weaving when she was 6—she only got as far as learning to twist the fibers into twine before she got discouraged and quit. This is her second time around and she has already thrown away three nets that began unsatisfactorily. There is only a limited exchange between mother and daughter and Sua seems more intent on finishing her own net than on pushing Nyenpu to finish hers. Nyenpu, for her part, frequently requests her mother's inspection, and spends a great deal of time just observing her mother's progress. Sua says that Nyenpu will not learn it this time (Plate 8.2) but next time, in perhaps a year, she will get it down. I was often told that it is a waste of time to attempt to help children learn "before they're ready." Had Nyenpu shown an interest in net weaving earlier, say at 4, Sua would have, in all likelihood, actively discouraged this interest.

Contrary to the impression created in Vygotskian-inspired research on "situated learning" (Rogoff & Lave, 1984), Sua does not scaffold or in-

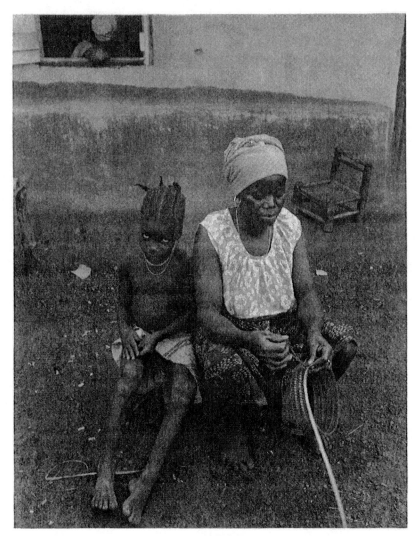

PLATE 8.1. Mother and daughter weaving fishnets.

terfere with Nyenpu's incipient net in any way. In that literature there is a great deal of emphasis on the role of the adult teacher, but, for the Kpelle, at least, the burden of skill acquisition rests almost totally on the learner (see also Greenfield & Lave, 1982, p. 183). Adults are willing to be observed and copied and, when asked, to serve as critic. But, the learner must have the maturity, intelligence, and perseverance or else there will be no situated learning (Rogoff & Lave, 1984).

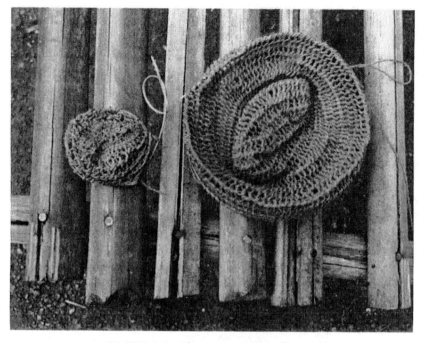

PLATE 8.2. Their respective efforts.

Sua started spinning cotton when she was 7 years old, but Nyenpu shows no inclination to learn this skill and Sua has no intention of teaching it to her. Girls wear beads strung on cotton thread. When she went to her mother for thread, Sua recalls being told, "It's time you learned to make your own." Or when a girl wanted new clothes, her mother would say, "Learn to spin and you'll get some clothes." So Sua started out with cornsilks, which she spun into thread; later she stole some of her mother's cotton and took it behind the house to practice spinning. A girl is expected to learn spinning on her own and if she is clumsy at it she will be teased. One common mistake is to spin the spindle toward rather than away from the waist and when Sua did this her mother would laugh at and smack her.

Chief Wollokollie's youngest wife, Goma, was an expert at *Bii paa*, or bag weaving (Plate 8.3). Goma had asked her big sister to teach her how to do it, but her sister refused so Goma taught herself. Now she is teaching a teenage girl of 16 how to do it. The girl has prepared the strands of palm leaf and brought them to Goma to help her get started. The two alternate at weaving the bag. The girl makes a mistake and Goma unravels what she

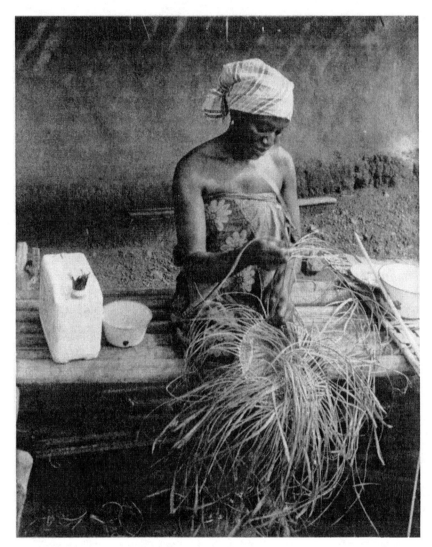

PLATE 8.3. Woman weaving bag.

has done, does it correctly for awhile, then lets the girl take over again. Goma can not explain how to do it, either to me or to the girl. She can only show and guide our hands as I, too, make an attempt to learn. It is not easy to learn and we make mistakes, but Goma is patient. She is partly rewarded by seeing a man, and a white man at that, doing woman's work, which is very amusing. Goma is the sort of patient teacher depicted in the

Vygotskian literature (Rogoff & Lave, 1984), but, as she herself pointed out, she is unusual; it is more common for "pupils" to be beaten for making mistakes or failing to pay attention.

Mat weaving is done almost exclusively by boys (Plate 8.4). Men without teenage sons may make their own mats or buy them. The size, quality, and quantity of woven mats varies directly with age, so that a boy of 9 may weave two to three mats in a year. These are generally small, about 1 meter × 1.6 meters, and they are of poor quality—the weft is not packed tightly and the edges are left unfinished causing the mat to fall apart in a short period of time. Boys actually begin mat weaving earlier than 9, but they do not weave functional mats. They take scraps left over from an older brother's mat and practice weaving them into small squares. They will watch the older brother as he weaves, fetching pieces for him, and, perhaps, if he gets up for a break, take his place and weave a line or two. The boys are not taught in any formal sense; they learn entirely through observation and imitation. By age 13, boys are weaving 10 or more large (2.3 meters × 2 meters) mats a year, and these are tightly woven with no holes and finished around the edges with a fiber braid. These

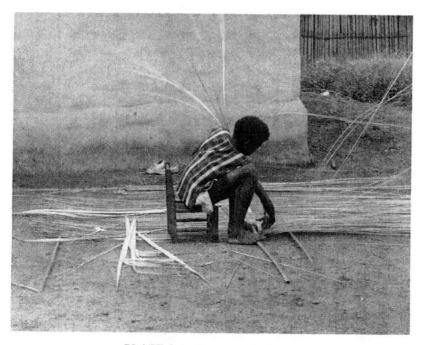

PLATE 8.4. Boy weaving mat.

mats are substantial and last a year or more. Speed and dexterity gradually increase so that an older boy can make a large mat in much less time
than the younger boy takes to make a small one. Another important
change is that older boys concentrate more fully on their task. A young
boy will start a mat, work on it for an hour or so, until some friends happen along, and go off to play. It may take him a week of sporadic work to
finish the mat. If his father needs the mat urgently, the father will finish it
himself. An older boy usually can finish a mat in 2 days; he works almost
without stopping, but he will chat with friends who stop by as he works.

Akewoli-la was 16 when he learned to weave a hammock; now he
makes about 10 a year which he gives to friends. When he was 16 he saw a
friend making a hammock. The friend asked Akewoli-la to help him, but
Akewoli-la protested that he did not know how. The friend offered to
teach him, at no charge. In a week, Akewoli-la went off to make his own.
It was very good and when he showed it to his teacher, the man jokingly
accused him of knowing how to do it all along. Now Akewoli-la is teaching
his son Tondolo (age 21) how to make a hammock. He teaches by demonstration, showing his son where to place and how to tie the knots.

Tondolo was anxious to make his own and did successfully with only
a few minor corrections by his father. He is now working on his second.
Every evening he spends about 2 hours twisting the fibers into twine and
nearly has enough, after 2 weeks, to make the hammock. Other hammock
makers reported that they first made miniature hammocks before making
a full size one. Apparently these individuals began learning it at an early
age, say, 12. I surmise that they did not have the patience to prepare
enough twine for a full-size one and were anxious to get into the actual
hammock construction.

Lave and Wenger (1991) identified a cultural routine that fits the
above cases very well—and also extends to apprenticeship (Chapter 9).
They call this legitimate peripheral participation. Essentially, they have
broadened the earlier conceptualization of Vygotskian theory. For example, the claim that all learning is social was taken to mean that learners
would always be assisted by those who are more skilled—a claim the
Kpelle material fails to substantiate. But there need not be an expert present to see the influence exerted by society on the learner. In each of the
previous cases, we see individuals acquiring weaving skills to enhance their
own social participation. As Sua indicates, if a *girl* wants to "look nice," to
match the appearance of *women*, she must learn the skills to dress and dec-
orate herself. In attempting to do so, she will be accorded the status of a
"legitimate peripheral participant." She may be supplied with materials

and someone competent may agree to model the skill and also to critique the fledgling product. Miniature tools may be supplied. Overall, the society will treat these initial forays with respect—at worst, mild teasing is employed.

Leis (1972) identifies yet another cultural routine that highlights the social nature of skill acquisition. Children often tackle a chore "in company" (Plate 8.5). While Ijaw girls weave mats or fishing traps, they "sit together on a verandah while they work. Adults approve of group projects

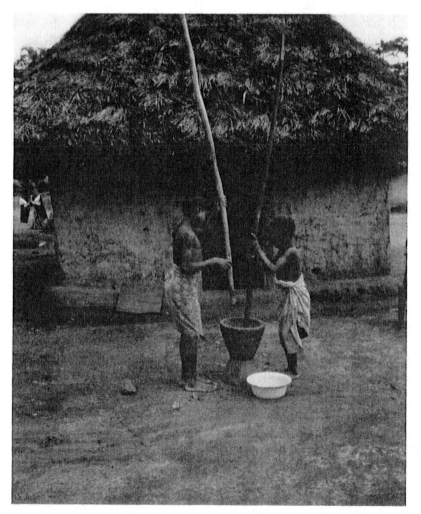

PLATE 8.5. Working in tandem.

because the girls work longer and learn more quickly helping each other than by weaving alone" (p. 53). In Gbangasuakwelle, children between 3 and 9 spend a great deal of the day in the company of members of their play group. But play groups also can function as work groups as the occasion warrants. I accompanied such groups on snail and mushroom gathering and water-, wood-, and bamboo-hauling expeditions.

MARKETING

Marketing (*Poni-too*), another area of the chore curriculum, is primarily done by men, but children also play a large role. They sell less expensive items such as shelled peanuts at 1 cent per *kopu* (plastic measuring cup, about 2 tablespoons in size). Small children (i.e., 5 to 7 years old) will carry a pan of peanuts on their heads around the town. They say nothing and do nothing, but because of their height, everyone can see what is on their heads. They are stopped by peanut buyers, usually older children, who first pay their penny then get a cupful of peanuts poured into their hands. They deeply distrust child buyers, who frequently grab handfuls without paying.

Children also sell palm nuts. A mother reaches into her woven bag and pulls out palm nuts picked by her husband. She lays them neatly on a woven tray and groups them by seven. After she has five groups, she places small sticks between the groups to set them apart. She calls her 7-year-old son and, placing the tray on his head, tells him to ask a penny for each set. He should bring back five pennies,[5] one of which is his to keep. He will walk around the town, where potential customers can see his wares. He may stand quietly by a group of men talking until they notice him, hoping to make a sale. When a customer indicates he wants to make a purchase, the boy lays down the tray and answers the question, "How much?" with "1 cent, 1 cent." The customer hands over 1 cent and takes one of the groups; the boy continues his rounds. He is not expected to make change. He verifies, by adding his accumulated pennies to the remaining piles, that he has not made a mistake. It should always total five. He does not lay his tray down to go and play because someone will steal his nuts. Nor does he spend the pennies, lest he get a beating (Plate 8.6).

Older children sell rice at 15 cents per cup, oranges at three for 5 cents, bananas at 1 cent each, papaya at 25 cents each, and so on. They can add and subtract, although it may take some time for them to figure out how much to charge for 17 bananas and how much change to give for

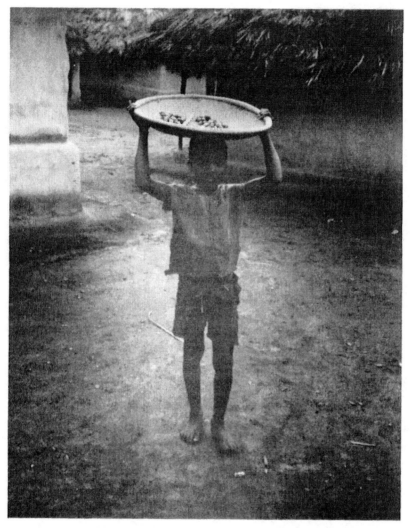

PLATE 8.6. Boy with tray of produce for sale.

a quarter. Some items that vary in size are open for bargaining (e.g., squash, tomatoes, eggplant, and cassava). In this case the child is not permitted to sell for less than the original price, but he may carry the item back to his mother with the buyer's offer and she will agree or send him back with a counteroffer. As Table 8.1 shows, one-third of the children at age 6 sell regularly and the percentage levels off to 80% by age 11.

Two factors allowed me to conduct fairly detailed observations of the selling process and to confirm repeatedly that very young sellers can not add and subtract: (1) I didn't have a garden, and (2) I had money so I attracted more than the usual amount of commercial traffic.

I questioned why children bear the major burden for daily selling[6] and the answer was interesting and reflective of the society's values. I was told frequently that to sell, one had to walk about the town and enter or look into people's houses to see if they were at home. If an adult male or female were to do this, he or she might be suspected of (1) adultery, (2) thievery, or (3) making *kpamo*, or black magic. Children are not susceptible to these faults (for a parallel case, see Schildkrout, 1990) so they can move about the town more freely. Again, referring to Table 8.1, boys, and especially young men, sell in the town more regularly than their female counterparts. This is because girls after age 11 are exposed to lewd remarks and advances when they travel alone through the town. When young women do sell, they usually go in pairs. Marketing can be devided into selling and trading. Selling would involve no bargaining, no planning or calculation of amount × price = total sale, all of which would be included in trading. Put this way, children "sell," whereas men and women "trade."

To return to the example of the palm nuts, what seems like a simple task is made possible only through the interaction of a variety of skills, all of which must be acquired before the boy is permitted to sell the nuts. From the age of 3, he has learned how to balance things on his head, starting out with a small, empty pan and proceeding to large, unwieldy loads weighing over 100 pounds, which he will carry as an adult. He has learned the concept of equivalence. Despite the fact that no two palm nuts are exactly alike, any two groups of seven are equivalent to each other and each can be exchanged for an equivalent value in cash (i.e., 1 cent). The concept is not fully formulated, however. He still has trouble with the fact that a 5-cent piece equals five 1-cent pieces.

He has been learning, since the age of 7, when his mother first let him roam around the town out of her sight, where groups are likely to gather in the town. So his journey through the town is purposeful and direct. He has observed, since at least the age of 2, that adults are powerful authority figures who can reward (1-cent tip) or punish (a beating). He has learned the value of sustained effort. He does not stop to play but rather perseveres until the task is completed.

How do adults know when children are "ready" for these assignments? Perhaps "there['s] a 'track' system of education to be found in nonliterate . . . societies" (Nerlove, Roberts, et al., 1974, p. 293). This study in Guatemala suggested that adults observe children at play and as they do simple chores, decide when they are "ready" for more challenging assignments, and also determine their talent and intelligence. Rogoff et al. (1975) also found, from an extensive review of the ethnographic literature, a widespread tendency to mark the transitions from early childhood (ages 5 to 7) and adolescence by assigning additional and/or new responsibilities.

By about 15, the Kpelle boy has achieved a degree of economic self-sufficiency. For example, whenever there is a teenage son in the family, he taps and sells palm wine, and there is a kind of tacit agreement that he's to take care of whatever needs he may have (i.e., clothing, cigarettes, and the favors of girls) out of the income from his palm wine and not to ask his father for money or goods. The pissava trees are tapped for the (naturally) fermented sap. Each tapper has his own working kit, which includes a special long-handled knife, a pan to catch the sap, and hollow gourds in which to transport it. The wine must be cleaned—cleared of a great deal of debris—before it is ready for sale. If the wine is tapped in the morning, the tapper walks around the town with his gourd of wine and a glass and, wherever he finds people gathered for work or talking matter, offers it to them at 5 cents a glass. If the wine is tapped in the afternoon, the tapper sits down in front of his house in the evening and calls out, "Come let's drink." His customers come to him, but now they buy the whole gourd (approximately a gallon at 70 cents) to take home. Of course, a tapper may drink his own wine, but he will sell most of it.

A teenage son may accompany his father on a trip to Gbarnga (the county seat) to sell his surplus rice. The Lebanese man in the general store on Main Street offers to buy the rice at $8.50 per bag. He carries the rice down to the mill. The government-run rice mill offers $8 a bag. He carries the rice back to the Lebanese man to conclude the sale.

But the process is not as simple as it seems, because the farmer must make many calculations and decisions beforehand. He must determine how large a farm to make in the first place so that he will have enough rice left over, after allocating some to each member of his family and setting some aside to use as seed rice for next year, to sell. He must sell enough to cover the cost of the government's imposed hut tax, any other fixed expenses he may have (brideprice payments, court fines) and variable expenses (medical). What is left over can be spent on luxuries. Once the rice is harvested, he allocates it. The portion that is to be sold is taken from the stalk and put into burlap bags. He now has several options. He can sell it to the local Mandingos, who grow no rice of their own. They might pay as much as $10 a bag, but only for hulled rice. Hulling that much rice takes time and labor. If he asks his wives to do it, they will expect a substantial portion of the hulled rice in payment.

Or, he can take it to Gbarnga and sell it unhulled. Although the father does not explain his decision-making processes to his son, after seeing the results of his father's decisions year after year, the son will naturally begin to acquire his own version of this process. He will not have a bag of rice of his own to sell for many years, but, in the intervening time, he will have sold bananas, palm wine, fresh game that he has trapped, and so on. The amount of money that goes through his hands gradually increases. The complexity of the selling process, making change, haggling over price, and trading for other goods is also increasing.

SUMMARY OF CHILDREN'S WORK

We interviewed all children in Gbarngasuakwelle between ages 6 and 13 and asked them what kinds of skills they felt they were competent in. Table 8.1 presents the results. Making market is one of the few skills practiced by boys and girls, and they begin at a very young age. Net weaving is exclusively a female task, whereas mat weaving, trap making, kitchen building, palm nut cutting, and palm wine making are almost exclusively male tasks. The critical age during which these tasks are at least attempted appears to be 9. The results also convey clearly that this is only approximately a "graded" curriculum. Unlike bush school and apprenticeship (see Chapter 9), which embody elements of formal education, skill acquisition in these areas is informal and depends a great deal on the motivation and persistence of the learners. No one gets upset if 12-year-old Togba can not make palm wine—he will not be labeled "learning disabled" and sent to special classes for remedial palm wine makers. No one will bother young Flumo for not doing his trap-making homework.

Other male tasks, not included in the questionnaire, are spoon carving, cloth weaving, and hammock weaving; basket weaving, fanner weaving, bag weaving, and spinning are female tasks. Medicine making is done by both sexes. Fish traps, kitchen baskets, and meat dryers are made by boys and old men. Unlike mats, however, these items are associated with luxury foods and are peripheral to the main food production. Boys and old men are in a similar position as far as food production is concerned. They do not make their own farms, yet they eat rice from someone's farm, which is, in effect, paid for by their gifts of woven items or the meat caught or stored in them.

TABLE 8.1. **Percentage of Children Who Practice Selected Types of Work**

Types of work	Age (yr)							
	6	7	8	9	10	11	12	13
Weave mats	0	0	46	83	40	92	50	100
Cut palm nuts	0	7	15	100	40	67	71	100
Make palm wine	0	0	0	42	33	75	71	100
Build rice kitchen	0	0	8	33	33	42	43	75
Weave nets	0	29	10	25	63	57	100	68
Marketing	32	43	68	76	65	79	90	73

Children learn three types of tasks at three different ages. They begin performing such rudimentary tasks of rice farming as cooking, pounding rice, and chasing away birds at a very early age, usually before they are 9. More difficult tasks, such as hoeing on the farm, net weaving, and trap making, are begun around age 9 and mastered by age 13. Rarer, more complex skills such as cloth weaving, bag weaving, blacksmithing, and medicine making are acquired in the late teens and may be learned after marriage.

Individuals learn various kinds of work in three educational processes, corresponding roughly to three age periods and three types of work. Children appear quite eager to take on and master chores they see their parents and older siblings engaged in. And they are rewarded and supported for doing so (Goodnow, 1988). On the other hand, the only time I ever saw parents get furious at their children was when the children refused or tried to avoid doing the simple tasks associated with rice farming and food preparation. The classic theories of learning and motivation (e.g., Skinner, 1963; White, 1959) account very well for children's learning during this stage. I would include all farmwork except palm work and tree planting in this stage, as well as fixing up the town, building things, and selling. This stage continues until the child is in his or her midteens and thus overlaps the next stage.

Somewhat later, around age 9, children may begin to learn more complex tasks, sometimes on their own and sometimes with the aid of an expert of the same sex. I say *may* because the performance of such tasks as net weaving and trapping is optional. Ideally the child will want to copy the same-sex parent and learn these skills, but, unlike farmwork, it is not mandatory. The child must want to learn and the parent, an older sibling, or another potential tutor may show some reluctance to teach the child until he or she demonstrates intense motivation to learn.[7] The child must still depend heavily on observing the expert's work and attempt to imitate it. Once he or she has made the attempt, however, the expert intervenes as teacher to correct mistakes, to offer advice, and to consciously "demonstrate" the skill. I would include spinning, all types of weaving except cloth weaving, tree planting, palm work, making medicine (other than medicines owned by *Zò-na*), wood carving, and trading in this stage.

There is a push–pull quality to the adult–child relationship. Adults force children to become increasingly independent by denying them choice foods (e.g., meat) and other valued resources. This is frustrating for children, but they are also moved by the desire to earn their own resources through their newly developing skills. The fact that these various skills are practiced out in the open means that children already have a good working model in their heads and they have a good idea where to find raw materials and what to do with them. Their initial attempts at mastery accomplish two things: They acquire some simple prerequisites and they demonstrate their commitment to their potential tutors.

The third stage, treated more fully in the next chapter, is associated with adolescence and young adulthood. Now the individual is exposed to information that is not public, that may be emotionally charged and secret. Or, there may be crafts whose complexity demands something more than observation and imitation, trial and error. The society tightens up its "entrance requirements" and its "curriculum." For certain kinds of information, conveyed during initiation rites, *everyone* in a particular age/cohort must participate. For other information (e.g., divination procedures), only one, favored individual may be selected for instruction. Teachers are so designated and instructional procedures are standardized. In a word, individuals are "schooled."

CHAPTER 9

Apprenticeship and Bush School as Formal Education

A child doesn't listen until it hurts.
—KPELLE PROVERB

The structure of an apprenticeship is very rigid and conservative. The apprentice is not expected to innovate, alter, change or improve upon anything. He is to copy the master's techniques . . . exactly.
—DEFENBAUGH (1989, p. 173)

In the previous chapter, I discussed the gradual and informal transition that occurs as a child or adolescent embarks on a mission to acquire a particular skill. These missions, although not solitary, are generally free of direct adult guidance or intervention. Indeed, if someone possesses a skill, especially a rare one, he or she is often reluctant to pass it on and will do so only to someone for whom he or she feels some affection or to someone who offers a big fee. So, what happens when the skill to be learned is so complex it cannot be acquired through observation, imitation, trial, and error? Again and again, societies have come to rely on a cultural routine we identify as "apprenticeship."[1] Further, we can ask what happens when a society decides that some aspects of its "moral" curriculum cannot reliably be acquired through the infomal means of play, songs, and observation/imitation? Many societies provide a sometimes extensive inititiation ceremony, which, in West Africa, has been referred to as bush school. This chapter compares apprenticeship and the bush school with our more formal methods of education (see also Lancy, 1975b).

LEARNING TO WEAVE AS AN APPRENTICE

Cloth weaving is far more complex than the weaving activities described in the previous chapter. When Chief Wollokollie was 22 he learned to weave from his older brother, who had, in turn, learned it from their father. Chief Wollokollie's experience closely resembled an apprenticeship. His brother wove cloth seven to eight times a year and each time Wollokollie learned an additional step in the operation. The first step he learned was preparing the warp. His brother watched and showed him how to wind the thread around the stakes and how to keep count. Then Chief Wollokollie learned to make the loom and for the next several weaving sessions he was in charge of preparing warp and loom. Then he learned to thread the heddles and reed (Plate 9.1) and, later, how to make his own. His brother taught him to sew the cloth strips together and Wollokollie did this chore as his brother wove the cloth. Finally, after 2 years of tutelage Wollokollie learned the actual weaving, with his brother dropping by frequently to check on his progress. Wollokollie made his brother an initial gift (white Kola) of a chicken, a bottle of palm oil, and three cups of rice. After he completed his training he gave his brother two of the ll-strip spreads he had woven.

Wollokollie remembered watching men weave from an early age. He watched his father weave and helped him fetch poles for the loom and when he was learning from his brother he watched the whole process intently. Similarly, among the Tukolor, another West African society:

> Boys brought up in weaving households begin to play around the loom at an early age. By the time they reach the age of ten or eleven years, boys have practiced most of the rudimentary tasks performed in the weaving shed, such as bobbin-winding, preparing shop-bought yarn on the bark, and even taking a turn at weaving on an apprentice's loom. . . . If he is the son of the weaver, the boy's play activities become more organized and he is integrated into the routine of the weaving shed. He is asked to wind bobbins for each weaver as needed, and now has a responsibility for completing his tasks thoroughly. His other duties are to undo and prepare hanks for rewinding, fetch water for the other weavers, and perform any other menial tasks that are required. (Dilley, 1989, p. 187)

However, "Some fathers prefer that another weaver should train their sons after they have acquired some basic skills during childhood, since they feel that they will not exert enough discipline in training" (Dilley, 1989, p. 188).[2]

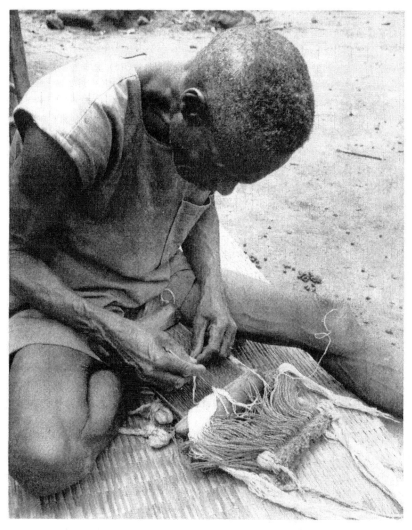

PLATE 9.1. Chief Wollokollie preparing to weave.

As with wood carving, the Kpelle are *not* noted for their cloth production, unlike several other West African societies in which cloth production is more refined and complex with a consequently lengthier and more demanding apprenticeship (Defenbaugh, 1989).[3] Also, among the Tukolor, "the . . . apprentice learns . . . not only the necessary skills in weaving . . . but also the mystical and religious aspects of craft lore" (Dilley, 1989, p. 190). This lore, for example consisted of verses "for weaving at incredible speeds . . . for weaving cloth . . . at the loom in one's absence" (Dilley, 1989, p. 196). This lore is called *gandal*. It includes the weaving origin myth and "can be used . . . to protect the weaver from spiritual forces associated with the craft and . . . as a means of defense against the malicious intention of other . . . weavers" (Dilley, 1989, p. 195). The Tukolor impose greater restrictions on access to weaving lore than on access to weaving skill per se. They "claim that a [nonmember] learning weaving lore would most certainly go blind or insane; the possession of lore is a symbol of exclusiveness of each craft[4] that provides a means of control over entry into it" (Dilley, 1989, p. 185).

Another aspect of the Tukolor apprenticeship that sets it apart as representing more *formal* education[5], is the levying of charges. "During the period of apprenticeship—about 3 years or more . . . the master . . . retains all the cloths the boy weaves, and takes the profit on them" (Dilley, 1989, p. 189). At the end of the apprenticeship, the boy and his parents make a prestation to the master who, in turn, gives the apprentice the moving parts of the loom. "The master may also present the youth with a small gift such as kola nuts as a reward for being attentive or as a restitution for the times the boy was beaten" (Dilley, 1989, p. 192).

THE CHARACTER OF THE APPRENTICE

Among the Kpelle, there appear to be only three areas of expertise that require the conduct of an apprenticeship: cloth weaving, blacksmithing, and medicine making (becoming a $Z\grave{o}$[6]). As few individuals in Gbarnga-suakwelle can claim to be expert at any of the three, this suggests a considerable degree of exclusivity. With the exceptional case of a twin singled out to become a $Z\grave{o}$ (Erchak, 1976/1977), no one is fated to become an apprentice. As we have seen, most Kpelle crafts are open to anyone with the motivation to learn them—as long as gender dimorphism is respected. For these three skills, individual motivation must be coupled with the willingness of the master to take on the individual as an apprentice. The apprenticeship also demands a degree of dedication well beyond that required to learn any other aspect of Kpelle culture. This also seems to be true of apprenticeship in other societies.

Singleton (1989) studied an apprentice learning from a Japanese master potter. "One Japanese term for apprenticeship is *minari*, literally one who learns by observation" (p. 14). There are five stages, including a prepractice stage, where the apprentice does menial tasks but no pottery work, and a postmastery stage, where the apprentice pays the master back by producing pottery for the workshop. Menial tasks could include, for example, turning the wheel, but the initial stage is primarily spent observing and soaking up the culture. Hence, "When an apprentice presumes to ask the master a question, he will be asked why he has not been watching the potter at work, or the answer would be obvious" (p. 26). On the other hand, just sitting around watching is discouraged; an apprentice must always be busy—working on clay, for example. The master conveys his evaluation by selecting a few of the apprentice's pieces for firing. Prior to this, all the apprentice's pots are destroyed or recycled.

It has been demonstrated empirically (Kaye & Giannino, cited in Greenfield & Lave, 1982) that learning via observation/imitation in contrast to trial and error or verbal instruction is very effective if the goal is to conserve traditional patterns but quite dysfunctional for producing innovation and improvement in technique or design.[7]

Strict discipline is easier to maintain if master and apprentice are, initially, strangers; however, the apprentice will become an integral member of the master's household. To go the distance—up to 10 years—the apprentice must consistently demonstrate "a single-minded, wholehearted dedication to the craft. . . . Talent is to be developed through persistence, it is not considered to be inherited or innate" (Singleton, 1989, p. 29). This rather haughty attitude on the master's part coupled with a lengthy period of servitude by the apprentice—who gets little praise and much abuse for his or her efforts—is widely reported in the literature.[8] It looks strange from our perspective where formal education, including schooling for a great variety of "trade" specializations, is virtually free. But, let us remind ourselves that in many societies, the kinds of skills learned in the apprenticeship may be rare and valuable; successful Japanese potters are wealthy—even by Japanese standards.[9] And skills of this sort are considered valuable commodities which must be purchased by the sweat of the apprentice's brow. Further, by making the apprenticeship very demanding and taking on few apprentices in one's career, the master ensures that there will be little competition so he can keep his prices high.[10]

For the Kpelle, the role of blacksmith carries with it such an annuity. The blacksmith's skills are in high demand and his social position is guaranteed by the pivotal role he plays in many ritual events. Not surprisingly, then, becoming a blacksmith in Gbarngasuakwelle requires a lengthy apprenticeship.

BECOMING A BLACKSMITH

Although the Kpelle failed to develop the rich wood-carving traditions of their neighbors, they *were* noted for their iron tools. According to Thomasson (1987), the Kpelle have a long history of mining the local iron ores and were quite sophisticated in the production of a rust-resistant alloyed metal. Nowadays, the Kpelle no longer work iron deposits, relying instead on scrap iron, and there is little intravillage trade in tools or iron money. However, within any town, the blacksmith does a lively business producing tools—such as the short-handled hoe and bushknife—not available from stores.

As illustrated in an earlier analysis (Lancy, 1980a), becoming a Kpelle blacksmith involves mastery of three distinct spheres. First, one needs to learn how to turn iron and wood into useful products. Second, because of his very public persona, his "extra" income, and the heavily symbolic nature of his craft, the blacksmith will inevitably assume the trappings of a "big man." The blacksmith's forge is one of the most popular male gathering points in town and the blacksmith is privy to a great deal of gossip and often consulted on legal, government, and social affairs. This is an awesome and dangerous responsibility, akin to that assumed by the town chief. Third, the blacksmith must also master the intricacies of the magicoreligious role of *Zò*, as he is often called on to conduct purifying rituals. The apprenticeship, per se, is straightforward, as we shall see. It is the other two spheres that involve many other cultural routines—including make-believe play—(Lancy, 1980a).

McNaughton (1988) apprenticed himself to a Mande (Mali—distantly related to the Kpelle) blacksmith, and he claims that "blacksmiths . . . in sub-Saharan Africa . . . are at once glorified and shunned, feared and despised" (p. xiii). "Clients often come to Sedu, to have old tools repaired or new tools made. But they also come with a request for soothsaying, amulet-making, medical diagnosis and treatment, and general advice on all kinds of problems" (p. xv). "Their anvils may be called upon to serve as the surface on which oaths or obligations are sworn" (p. 65).

I was unable to observe an apprenticeship in progress, so I interviewed both of the blacksmiths working in Gbarngasuakwelle to get their retrospective memories.

> Jaiwo-Gbala was apprenticed to his mother's brother. At first he only helped out on occasion by bringing wood for the forge and by operating the bellows. But even before this, Jaiwo remembers sitting on a log at one end of the

"shop" and watching his uncle work. At 14 he began a formal apprentice-ship that lasted three years. his father "gave" him to his uncle; then, at the end of the apprenticeship, the uncle "gave" him back to his parents. Jaiwo-Gbala first learned to make a knife blade, then a machete; later still he learned to carve wooden handles and to forge the hoe and the adze. These latter two require bending the hot iron, which must be done with care to avoid breaking it. His uncle made few comments while Jaiwo-Gbala was working; only when he had finished a tool would he give a detailed critique. He was not allowed to keep a piece until it was perfect, nor could he make a machete until he had mastered the knife, a hoe until he had mastered the machete, and so on. When he made a mistake or did sloppy work, his teacher would beat and berate him and order him to destroy what he had made. During the apprenticeship, he paid his uncle through his work. He would make tools for people who would, in turn, agree to work on his uncle's farm. The apprenticeship terminated when Jaiwo-Gbala had mas-tered all the tools, including those needed in the actual blacksmithing, and he set up his own forge.

Yakpawlo, the second of the two blacksmiths in Gbarngasuakwelle, was "adopted" by his teacher. When he was eight he went with his father and a group of men to bring back a big rock for the blacksmith to use as an anvil. The smith saw him, liked him, and, not having a son of his own, asked Yak-pawlo's father for him. he lived with the smith until he was grown and ready to start his own forge. He too began by working the bellows, graduated to fix-ing old machetes and knives, and then to fabricating whole tools. When his apprenticeship was complete at 18, his father gave the smith 48 armspan lengths of cloth, two chickens, and a goat. Yakpawlo worked for both his fa-ther and the smith until they died; that is, he shared part of his payments with them. (Lancy, 1980a, pp. 269–270)

Both men indicated that their masters had berated and beaten them when they made mistakes. Coy (1989), another anthropologist/appren-tice blacksmith, mentions this and also indicates the use of a kind of "fi-nal exam": At the end of the apprenticeship he was given an iron rod and told to turn into a spear. McNaughton (1988) notes that the appren-tice works with a scaled-down set of tools, initially. For the Mande the apprenticeship lasts 7 to 8 years of very hard work. The apprentice must work the bellows for hours. It is hot, tiring, and boring; boredom may be relieved by playing simple rhythms on the bellows. Not surprisingly, some apprentices quit.

Before the apprentice works with metal, he must learn to select the proper wood for handles and to cure it. He learns to carve the handles. Al-though the master is present, he "rarely stop[s] work in progress, preferring to let the lad discover his own mistakes" (McNaughton, 1988, p. 28). The apprentice is expected to watch, to ask, but is never given unsolicited advice. Then, late in the apprenticeship, the novice is introduced to what I have earlier referred to as lore. This includes sorcery (snake handling and divination with cowries) and folk medicine. He learns to make amulets: "There are hundreds of different kinds of amulets, each designed for a specific function" (McNaughton, 1988, p. 58).

To conclude this section, I will briefly reexamine skill acquisition in light of a review of the skills learned via apprenticeship. Figure 9.1 illustrates the relationship among a number of factors we have been considering. It shows, for example, that as the particular skill becomes more complex, it is pursued by only a few of the older children or adolescents. Most skills fall along a neat continuum where learning difficulty is positively correlated with age and negatively correlated with the number of active practitioners. Many skills are discrete, and the distinction between practitioner and nonpractitioner is clear. However, selling and farmwork are dynamic; all individuals seem to gradually acquire a more sophisticated version of these skills as they grow older.

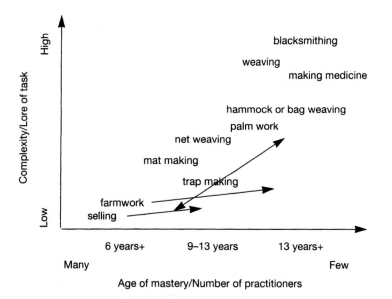

FIGURE 9.1. Relationship between skill complexity, age of acquisition, and number of practitioners.

BUSH SCHOOL

Although descriptions of childhood are rare in the ethnographic literature, the rites of passage into adolescence are widely noted.[11] Erny (1981) complains: "Many observers, especially among the earliest, have created the impression that traditional African education can in fact be reduced to pubertal initiation" (p. 139). An obvious explanation is that, to this point, enculturation has been achieved through the subtle effect of informal cultural routines (e.g., games) and are, thus, likely to be overlooked. Initiation rites are not only formal, they usually involve fantastic ritual of some sort (meat and potatoes for the field anthropologist). Also, these rites, sometimes referred to as bush school, are the closest analogue to our own public schooling. So, bush school is noticeable and, seemingly, familiar. On the other hand, it is also shrouded in secrecy. Hence, ethnographic descriptions, although common, tend to be rather spotty. This is certainly true for the Kpelle. I will attempt to build a composite picture based on the work of several Kpelle ethnographers, work with such closely related tribes as the Mende, and other studies from Africa and Papua New Guinea.

In Chapter 6, I introduced *Bambé*, a young boys' version of an adult secret society, complete with initiation, secrets and medicine. Somewhat more elaborate still is *Gbliŋ Gbe*:

> . . . a mock association for young boys. They participate before joining the *Poro*. Although there are no medicines that belong to the society, they do practice chicken sacrifices. The boys grab chickens that are wandering about the town, take them into the bush, kill them in a sacrificial manner, and eat them. If caught, they're not punished provided they can establish that their activities were part of the *Gbliŋ Gbe*. The boys choose one of their number to act as the *Zò* and another as the *bakuŋ*, or assistant. After their sacrificial meal they go about the town in a processional, copying the behavior of their fathers in the regular societies. In this manner, the boys learn what it is like to belong to the major [secret] societies and get their first experience with having to practice a version of the secrecy proscription. (Bellman, 1983, pp. 37–38)

This suggests that boys have some knowledge of what is in store for those who are initiated and some desire to acquire the trappings and enhanced status of inititiands.

But, there must also be great trepidation, as well. Chodorow (1978) found a near universal tendency to see the attainment of manhood as questionable due to boys' attachment to the mother and women's influence during childhood. As noted in Chapter 5, children stay attached to their mother's back or breast throughout a long infancy and sleep with her until they are weaned at 3 to 4 years of age. The child grows up in a household in which there may be several adult women, but the lone adult male, who heads the household, may spend little time in the "bosom" of the family and is not expected to have much to do with children. Hence, male initiation is often a violent rending of the Oedipal bond.

Erny (1981) notes that "among the Hero, the boys used to arrive for circumcision dressed in feminine clothes, finery and jewels in order to show that they were still carriers of a partly feminine nature" (p. 150). For the Ibo, "the initiation symbolically separates the boy from his mother, the child returning home a different social and psychological person. . . . The breaking of the calabash, a symbolic uterus . . . , marks the . . . end of the gestation period" (Ottenberg, 1989, pp. 189–190). For the Bena-Bena, "initiation has to do with ridding the initiates of any trace of feminine character or influence while at the same time maintaining power and control over females and the power of procreation" (Langness, 1981, p. 22). Little (1970) reports for the Mende, northeastern neighbors of the Kpelle, that the violent and bloody cicatrization of initiates is accompanied by a "'spirit' [who] plays loudly on his pipe and there is a clapping of hands, which drowns the noise of the boys' cries and prevents them being overhead by passers-by, especially women and children" (p. 214).

It must be difficult for mothers to accede to this process. In Kpelle villages, they make a valiant effort to prevent their boys from being taken. Bellman (1983) describes bush school as "a kind of theatrical play" (p. 112), suggesting that the women are playing a well-rehearsed role.[12] In the "separation" phase of the typical rite of passage (van Gennep, 1909/1960), the initiates,[13] *Kpulu nuu*, are

> captured, terrified, from their huts, and hurled over a thatch fence in the sacred *Poro* grove in the forest. On the other side of the wall, terrible frightening sounds can be heard. Once over, the boys are surrounded by fearsome masked and costumed figures, ancestral spirits, called "devils" in English. One of them holds each boy while another carves deep cuts in a design on his back, chest, and stomach. The cuts are treated to make them swell and heal in permanent raised scars. This pattern of cicatrization . . . entitles each man to attend and participate in *Poro* ritual anywhere, even in the territory of non-Kpelle. (Erchak, 1992, p. 68)

At the onset, boys are given wooden swords dipped in chicken blood and sent to fight the devil Namu. They inevitably are defeated and "eaten"—the cicatrization scars represent teeth marks—and live in the belly of the devil until they are later reborn. After this initial, dramatic separation stage (cf. van Gennep, 1909), the men return to town from the bush; on the way, they "stop and pick a particular leaf that contains a red latex that signifies the blood of the initiates" (Bellman, 1983, p. 81).

As ties with the mother are severed, these rites also serve to assert the authority of men (Spencer, 1970). Among the Sambia, for example, fathers are excluded lest they attempt to mitigate the child's suffering (Herdt, 1990). Ngoni boys are removed from their homes to live in a kind of dormitory to (1) remove them from women's influence, (2) build solidarity in the warrior class, and (3) make them more readily subordinate to elders. "Ngoni . . . fathers . . . expected [dormitory living] to produce toughness, leadership, responsibility and respect for authority" (Read, 1960, p. 94). In some cases, this respect must be coerced, as indicated by the proverb in this chapter's epigram. A boy who has been "frisky" is given "especially painful scarification" (Bellman, 1983, p. 112). A Sambia "lad tries to run away but is grabbed; as a punishment he is next bled harder and longer than the others" (Herdt, 1990, p. 376).

North Central New Guinea seems to represent an extreme in terms of the severity of initiation, and the range of tactics employed by the initiators would rival the Gestapo. In all these cases (Herdt, 1990; Hogbin, 1970b; Langness, 1981; Whiting, 1941) being manly means collaborating in an undertaking to maintain enmity between men and women; to maintain men's subjugation of women, "men are in full charge of public affairs; women are relegated to heavy, dirty garden work" (Herdt, 1990, p. 369). Further, the initiation process represents preparation for warrior status. A leader, perhaps a respected shaman or a warrior, lectures to young men about women's pollution and the glory of warfare.

Following their dramatic initiation, life in Kpelle bush school settles into a routine that lasts quite a long time, ideally 4 years for boys and 3 for girls. This is the transition or isolation phase common to rites of passage (van Gennep, 1909/1960). The boys live in a special village erected in the *Poro* section of the bush. The whole affair is managed by the *Zò-na*,[14] each of whom has different responsibilities. Although there is some suggestion that boys are "taught" in a manner analogous to Western schooling (Dennis, 1972), Ottenberg's (1989) assessment of the Ibo situation is more typical: "Formal education in the initiations is minimal, as it is only occasionally desirable in everyday Afikpo life. There really is no 'school in the bush,' the specific knowledge that the boys acquire is not extensive" (p. 237). Rather, the emphasis seems to be on the shaping of identity, indoctrination rather than education (Lancy, 1975b).

For the Kpelle, both boys and girls, bush school should impart a healthy respect for the *Ƶò-na*, their medicines, and magic. They learn the doctrine of *ifa mo*. And they learn that the "*contents* of the secrets are not as significant as are the *doing* of the secrets" (Bellman, 1983, p. 17). The omnipresence of the *Ƶò-na* also suggests a curriculum centered on lore and "Kpelle *wo su Bela* . . . 'deep Kpelle' . . . [which] includes extensive use in conversation of parables, metaphoric expressions, dilemma tales, and mythical narratives" (Bellman, 1983, p. xii).

> Finally, we have the third, incorporation, phase of the rite of passage. At the closing of bush school the general secrets are revealed, the secular identities of the masked figures are learned, and the boys take a solemn oath to uphold Poro and to never disclose its secrets, under pain of death. The boys don special raffia skirts, a symbol of their new manly status, and apply white clay to their skin, a symbol of their spiritually charged liminal state. When they triumphantly dance through the village at the end of their long, trying ordeal, they are older, more confident, have new names, and behave very differently, especially toward their mothers; they are men. They are symbolically reborn as men, having been killed as little boys. (Erchak, 1992, p. 68)

The material on boys' induction into *Poro* is sketchy, but girls' bush school experience and induction into *Sande* is largely unrecorded.[15] It appears to be broadly similar, however. Girls are also taken into a special area of the bush—ownership alternates between *Poro* and *Sande*—and they are "eaten" by a devil called *Ƶèɣele*. They are cicatrized and these scars, a permanent sign of *Sande* membership, are treated as teeth marks. Their isolation lasts 3 years and they are also reincorporated into society with much fanfare and a new name. Again, all this is managed by *Ƶò-na*, female rather than male, except for the presence of the head *Ƶò* of the *Poro* and the ubiquitous blacksmith. According to Bledsoe (1980), "the main purpose of *Sandi* rituals is to confer fertility on young female initiates" (p. 59). Also, Kpelle rationalize clitoridectomy—usually a part of *Sande* initiation—as removing a girl's friskiness and making her "more easily controlled by her husband" (Erchak, 1977, 127).

Audrey Richards's (1956) account of *Chisungu*, the women's bush school of the Bemba, a tribe inhabiting present-day Zimbabwe, is a classic study. *Chisungu* inculcates in these women an appreciation of Bemba beliefs about, for example, the magical potency of sex, fire, and blood. In this case we have a matrilineal society in which men are dominant, which creates a great deal of ambiguity that the puberty ritual helps to "explain." *Chisungu* is 6 months long, punctuated by semipublic ceremonies and rituals. There are various talismans made and distributed, and special songs are learned (more than fifty) during lengthy periods of dancing. "Each woman began to snatch at a *mufungo* bush for leaves . . . [which] they folded into cones to resemble small conical fish traps. They sang a song about setting fish traps and . . . pretended to catch each others fingers in the leaf traps" (Richards, 1956, p. 65). This is a humorous parable representing fertility. The traps and fingers represent the female and male sexual organs and a song with the repeated verse, "The fish has many children and so will the girl," is sung.

Through these songs and ceremonies the young woman is ritually indoctrinated into her role. There are references to gardening, parenting, and sexual intercourse. Women are also introduced to Bemba notions of personhood; for example, one clay figure made during the *Chisungu* "was a figure of a man with a large head and phallus and no arms. It represents a man who stays in the house all day finding fault with his wife and doing no work" (Richards, 1956, p. 103). A clay figurine of a hyena is introduced with the admonition, "The girl is not to steal like the hyena" (Richards, 1956, p. 105).

Like Bledsoe (1980) on the *Sande* bush school, Richards also discusses whether there is any direct instruction of a practical nature taking place during *Chisungu*:

> Rites representing hoeing, sowing, cooking, gathering firewood . . . occurred throughout the ceremony. But, instruction, in the European sense, was quite unnecessary in such subjects. Bemba girls play at cooking as soon as they can stand, and they help their mothers in the house most of the day. They go with the older women to garden and also learn from them how to look for [wild plants]. . . . The more complex aspects of housekeeping such as the care of the granary and reaping of grain are not introduced to the girl until some years after marriage. . . . Girls are not ignorant of the nature of sex . . . they have also acted as nurses of their young [siblings] . . . and are therefore familiar with the elements of the rather simple system of childcare practiced in this tribe. . . . The Chisunga teaches, not the technical activities of the wife, mother and housewife, but the socially approved attitude towards them. (pp. 126–128)

Ultimately, bush schools are extremely conservative, much more akin to "finishing schools," in our terms, than public schools. They reinforce the status quo, particularly, the power of men and of high-ranking men and women. Many, if not all, the messages conveyed in bush school have been heard before, but recall the point made about redundancy in Chapter 2. Whereas the earlier messages were embedded, perhaps, in folktales, now they are made more explicit. And, as Erny (1981) reminds us: "When it is a question of making important truths sink in, a physical or emotional shock is used in order to impress the individual, and thus increases receptivity" (p. 143). The bush school hammers home a few simple themes in an organized, ritual fashion. Unlike every other routine for enculturating children considered in this book, bush school is *compulsory*: "Anyone who is not a graduate of these schools is not considered human" (Dennis, 1972, p. 142). Furthermore, "Should a non-member accidentally witness [the] devil or the [secret] society's activities . . . he allegedly will either die, become blind, or suffer leprosy" (Bellman, 1983, p. 29).

THE INFORMAL–FORMAL EDUCATION CONTINUUM

A prominent theme in the cross-cultural literature on child development is the analysis via comparison/contrast of the learning environment of the school versus the village (Scribner & Cole, 1973). This analysis has been motivated in large part by concern for the low success rate of children from village backgrounds in Western-style public schools. The standard argument contrasts the informal patterns of instruction found in the village with more formal patterns found in school. I have argued (Lancy, 1975a, 1975b) for a modification of this dichotomy in pointing out both informal aspects of instruction in newly established Liberian rural public schools, on the one hand, and formal aspects of instruction in the traditional village curriculum (Lancy, 1980a), on the other.

A recent discussion (Greenfield & Lave, 1982, p. 183) provides a useful table of paired contrasts between formal and informal education. I have adapted and expanded their scheme and applied it to the Kpelle material in Table 9.1. However, a major difference in our thinking (see also Studstill, 1979) is that Greenfield and Lave tend to treat the school as the exclusive representative of the formal category, whereas I consider apprenticeship and initiation quite formal. In another area of disagreement, Greenfield and Lave suggest that in informal education, the "maintenance of continuity and tradition are valued" (p. 183) whereas in formal education, "change and discontinuity are valued" (p. 183). I believe just the opposite to be true in some cases. From the standpoint of the governing body, formal education can be very conservative. One of the prime rea-

TABLE 9.1. Kpelle Routines for Enculturation Reviewed from the Perspective of Informal versus Formal Education

Informal education (Chapters 5–8)	Formal education (Chapters 9 and 10)
The child's learning is somewhat incidental, it occurs, "naturally," in the course of daily activity. We see this happening with the "chore curriculum" (Chapter 8) and in the learning that takes place as children observe and imitate adults (Chapter 5).	In formal education, learning activities are set apart from the routine. The apprenticeship is set off spatially and temporally as is the initiation rite.
Children, themselves, must initiate learning opportunities. Their drive to become competent and their inherent curiosity leads them to experiment with adult skills (also, Chapters 5, 8).	The initiation rite is *compulsory*. Whereas one must volunteer for an apprenticeship, it represents a formal commitment to the educational process—a commitment sealed with the payment of fees. Especially where one has had support from one's kin to engage in the apprenticeship, great social pressure is exerted to ensure that one sees it through.
Anyone with a skill or knowledge can be a teacher at any time.	Specific individuals—the master blacksmith, the *Zò-na*—serve as teachers. That is, they hold both the knowledge and the authority of a "teacher." One can not learn these "secrets" on one's own or pick them up from acquaintances.
One's teachers are one's relatives and playmates (Chapter 6). This is somewhat of a mixed blessing—teachers are all around, but they may not have the time, energy, or patience to serve that purpose. They are as likely to provide obstacles as incentives for the ambitious child.	These teachers usually have few personal ties to the students. One reason for this is the perceived need to impose severe discipline, including corporal punishment.
The curriculum is mostly implicit and indirect. With make-believe (Chapter 5), games (Chapter 6), and stories (Chapter 7), children learn about important aspects of their culture through play.	The curriculum is quite explicit. There are stages or steps, lessons, tests, and induction and graduation exercises.
Observation and imitation are relied on very heavily. Occasionally—as with the learning of such skills as mat weaving and trap making (Chapter 8)—the teacher carefully demonstrates the construction process.	Formal teaching methods—where the teacher actually focuses complete attention on the learner—predominate. There is demonstration, explanation, and recitation which students must internalize and recapitulate. The atmosphere is more verbal.
The learner's primary motivation is to have fun interacting with peers and caretakers. Also, newly acquired skills may serve as social capital. Third, perhaps, the learner acquires cultural capital in the broad mastery of the "story" of the society (see also D'Andrade, 1984, p. 98).	The learner's motives tend to be quite explicit. Completion of bush school moves one up the status hierarchy—marriage, one's own plot of farmland, membership in secret societies, a house of one's own, motherhood, and so on. A successfully completed apprenticeship usually has immediate, positive monetary implications.

sons that societies go to the trouble of creating formal educational institutions is to preserve the "canon," so to speak. On the other hand, we have much evidence (Chapter 10) to suggest that children and adolescents in play can be quite innovative (Lancy, 1980b).

Although we can see many distinct contrasts between formal and informal education within the village, the difference between village education (including bush school) and public schooling is far greater than any contrast among cultural routines within the traditional society. When a child from the third world enters a Western-style public school, he or she is, indeed, entering a "Brave New World." This contrast is greatest along a dimension not included in the Greenfield and Lave (1982) table, namely, that between education and indoctrination. Bush school lasts, for Kpelle boys, 4 years, yet there is wide consensus that few skills and little information is imparted during this period; it is largely indoctrination. Likewise, we see outsiders mastering traditional crafts in a fraction of the time normally allocated to a traditional apprenticeship. Thus, although such areas as Kpelle medicine and blacksmithing may demand a level of information acquisition requiring a more formal approach with a structured curriculum and teachers, nothing in Kpelle society demands the acquisition of so much information in such a compressed time span as the typical public school curriculum. This dimension, of information mastered per unit of time, is perhaps the most critical contrast between informal and formal education and accounts, in large part, for the great difficulty Kpelle children have when they elect to travel down the *Kwii* road.

For Kpelle children, the "press" to acquire new, critical information is much greater in the public school than in the village. But the gap between school and home is not always this wide (Lancy, 1989). I remember clearly as a child, my father assigning me "extra" homework because my school curriculum seemed to him—raised in the classical European intellectual tradition—shallow and undemanding. Elsewhere (Lancy, 1983), I demonstrated a relationship such that children who have to acquire a great deal of information in becoming competent members of their society—as in a maritime foraging and trading society—will be advantaged as pupils in the public school. However, although apprenticeship and initiation may be found lying closer to the formal end of the continuum than other cultural routines, it is indeed rare that a society finds it must invent the peculiar routine that we take so much for granted. And when it does, this "school" will be used for only a very limited purpose.

CHAPTER 10

The Kwii Way

[Public education has led to] . . . an avalanche of failed aspirations
throughout the third world. . . .
—LEVINE AND WHITE (1986, p. 193)

Although Gbarngasuakwelle was isolated and a repository of much traditional Kpelle culture, signs of change were[1] evident. The term that symbolizes change to the residents of Gbarngasuakwelle is *Kwii*. It derives from Portuguese, the earliest white men to touch West Africa. Today, Lebanese traders are called *Potokwii*. They, like the earlier Portuguese, are white, exploitative outsiders. *Kwii* refers not only to people but to Western ideas and artifacts in general.

KWIINESS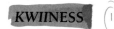

The thing that best symbolized change to the residents was a new road built by then President Tolbert to provide access to his upcountry estate. The road skirts the edge of town and was viewed literally as a medium of communication, channeling *Kwii* people, ideas, and artifacts into the town. Before there was a road *Kwii* was only talked about; with its completion—even though it was rarely traveled—*Kwii* became an ever-present phenomenon, injecting change and controversy into the town. In addition, while I was resident in Gbarngasuakwelle, the government sent an earnest young man to the town to begin holding classes (in English) to teach the Liberian standard curriculum.

To gauge people's reaction to change I conducted an open-ended interview with several adult informants. I asked them, first, what good things the road had brought, then what bad things.

179

SEYE-WULO (male): First, education, if you have that no one will ever scare you. Way back, it took a month to walk from here to Monrovia, so the vehicle has saved us trouble. Hospital. They used to cut sand for us, mosquito suck us, malaria makes us tremble. They said this is caused by spirit. Now they give you injections.

PAYE (male): We have fire to wrap up and put in our pocket and it doesn't know us, but when we are hungry we light it [matches].

SEYE-WULO: We know *Kwii* from "book." The way to tell a *Kwii*, his speaking English, his behavior, his clothing, the way he treats other people, he is clean, but the important thing is clothes and cleanliness.

PAYE: You two [I and my assistant] are *Kwii*.

NYANNI (male): *Kwii* people ask you for palm wine, you say you don't have any. They will beat you. Even if you can't read and write, if you are appointed by the government you are *Kwii*, you have power.

LORPU (male): The bad thing is, they take money from you, they take rice from you, they force you to work. This all comes from the government. This is bad *Kwii*. If they tell you to pay hut tax and you go and give your palm kernels, but they can force you to work for another man. If you have chickens or other animals in the town, they come and grab it.[2] Sometimes when a big person comes to see you, you offer him a chicken, but *Kwii* people just come and take them.

PAYE: The worst thing about *Kwii* is lawyers. Lawyers are ruining this country. I don't have money to hire a lawyer, but *Kwii* people do. These lawyers ruin my matter; how can I fight them. If they tell me now, go to Gbarnga, even if I don't have a lantern, I'll go in the darkness, suppose a snake is on the road, it will probably bite me. I must go, what can I do. Because they say, I must go and they will bring trouble on me if I don't go. Who will feed me there? I will be hungry.

SUA (female): The road has brought schools, we're able to sell our crops now, the road has brought white people, vehicles, zinc roofs, clothes. Before the road, if the baby shits on the mat, this mess will get on everyone, but now with kerosene lantern, flashlight you can see it and clean it up. Stealing, now we must put locks on our doors where before we didn't even know locks. Men come here and rape our women.

It is clear that people welcomed the technical improvements but strongly resisted the preemptory attitudes of the *Kwii* intruders. A case study illustrates the dimensions of the problem. One man in the village, universally despised as being lazy, sold land to a Mandingo man. The

Mandingo man cleared the land, preparatory to planting crops. In the process he cut down about an acre of cocoa trees that had been planted by another man, not the owner. This other man sued the Mandingo for damages. The town chief found against the Mandingo but he refused to pay, so the other man carried the matter to the District Commissioner in Gbarnga, the county seat. The District Commissioner found that the Mandingo owned legal title to the land and therefore could keep it and should pay only a token $3 in damages. The other man was still unsatisfied and threatened to destroy any crops the Mandingo man should plant. The District Commissioner agreed to send representatives to Gbarngasuakwelle to determine the extent of the damage so that an equitable settlement could be made. A month later three vehicles arrived in the town bearing the County Commissioner, an American working for the United Nations Development Project, the County Agriculture Agent, and assorted other officials, drivers, and hangers-on—about 15 people. Before they would inspect the damages they demanded food and drink. It was the officials' first visit ever to Gbarngasuakwelle even though it is one of the largest towns in the county. They complained bitterly about having to spend time in this out-of-the-way place and demanded special foods for their sensitive palates. After nearly 2 hours of eating and drinking, the County Commissioner demanded $17 from each litigant before the officials would inspect the field. The money was paid, the damage was assessed (although later, none of the 15 people could remember just how many of the cocoa trees had been cut down), and the Mandingo man was ordered to pay $150. They piled into their vehicles and left. The Mandingo man did not have $150, and the man who sued him had no power to force him to pay so the matter ended there. Neither party was satisfied, but both were at least $35 poorer as a result of the litigation.

This type of land dispute was becoming increasingly common because no one really owns land, yet residents can not resist selling land when an outsider makes an offer. The outsider, however, then takes out a deed to the land. Usually, land disputes are settled within the family, so to speak, but with title deeds and property lines, a claimant must now take his case to the government, which only exacerbates the problem.

This example and the interview reinforce many of my impressions in talking to residents about the road and change. In fact, I became the focus of many heated discussions because I was a tangible example of *Kwii*-ness—the color of my skin, my clothing, my taste in food and music, the strange things I did that I called work, and so on. Reactions ranged from the bemused wonderment of an old man like Yɛlɛkɛ, who knew that the changes he saw would never affect him very deeply and hence he could watch and learn about them in a detached manner, to the fiercely conservative Akewoli-la, who reacted against nearly all *Kwii* things with venomous distaste, to Monroe Kollie, who zealously nurtured his own nascent *Kwii*ness by attending school, talking English whenever he could, copying my behavior, and so forth.

CHANGES IN WORK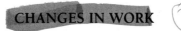

There had been few changes in the central work activity, rice farming. No labor-saving devices, no new technology, no changes in the division of labor here. Even the outsiders buying up land around the town plant it in rice, although they pay for the services of a *kuu* rather than working on *kuu* members' farms themselves. At various times, Liberia has had to import more than 50% of its staple and has a dismal history of expensive, failed schemes to increase rice production—a story repeated throughout Africa (Nsamenang, 1992). As Edgerton (1992) notes, "Folk populations typically adopt strategies that assure a life-sustaining but well below maximal yield of food and resist changes that entail what they perceive to be risks even though these new food-providing practices would produce more food" (p. 200).

Rice was, however, increasingly being used as a cash crop to raise money for the hut tax and for luxury items. This means larger farms and some supplementing of the diet with such introduced crops as yams, edoes, and peanuts. It is difficult to date just when a crop was first introduced into Gbarngasuakwelle, but there seemed to be a gradual shift taking place from group farmwork peculiar to rice growing to the more solitary labor associated with planting such things as coffee, cocoa, rubber, and garden crops.[3]

Fishing was dropping off as dried ocean fish was imported into town by Mandingos and sold at little stalls. Hunting was on the decline as wild game became scarce and domestic poultry and livestock became more plentiful.

The demand for skilled work was sharply declining. Plastic sandals, hats, and bags were replacing hand-made leather ones. Imported dry goods replaced hand-woven products because these were cheaper and more colorful. Machine-milled wood products replace hand-carved ones, and so on. All these changes point to a shift to a cash economy. The weaver no longer plants cotton and his wife and children no longer spin thread. Rather, they invest their time in cash cropping and use the returns to purchase imported cloth. An adolescent boy works on the president's estate at $1 per day. Twenty-five cents "buys" him the same amount of food he would have earned working on his father's farm, but now he has 75 cents left over to invest in clothes or earrings for his girlfriend. So fathers must use coercion to keep their children at work. Women sue their husbands for divorce, saying, "He never buys me anything." Providing food, shelter, and clothing was no longer sufficient to keep a wife happy and faithful. Jealousies and rivalries among co-wives were intensified as husbands now could purchase more tangible evidence of their preferences.

Changes in medicine making were proceeding at a more relaxed pace. Unlike other forms of work, medicine is buttressed by complex ritual and by the many secret societies. People were still getting sick and dying and belief in witchcraft and sorcery remained strong. People quickly adopted foreign medicines, but these were seen as supplementing rather than substituting for the traditional medicines. Even in the capital city of Monrovia, traditional medicine flourished and tribal beliefs and practices in this realm seem to have been thoroughly diffused into the modern sector of the country.

The doctrine of *ifa mo*, which permeates traditional medicine and the secret societies, has the effect of protecting these customs and beliefs from outside scrutiny and interference. A couple of my informants had achieved a grade-school education and made no attempt to hide their contempt for the traditions of their parents. Nevertheless, none of these young men was willing to discuss any details of his bush school or *Poro* experiences. And when students from Cuttington College in Gbarnga were to play a soccer game against a team from the University of Liberia, they pooled their money to purchase medicines from the *Zò-na* to ensure their rival's defeat.

In the area of medicine making, none of the young boys I talked to indicated any desire to become a *Zò*. They condemned many aspects of traditional medicine, especially the witchhunting societies, as "just fooling the people." Two boys said they might join the snake (*Kali-sali*) society because they could then *earn money* by curing snake bites. No young men were learning to weave and no young girls were learning to spin during my stay in the town, The children would rather buy cloth in the store. Both the blacksmith and the leatherworker expressed the strong desire to pass on their skills to a young man, preferably one of their sons, but none seem interested in learning. I asked these men why they did not force their children to work with them. They explained that to learn a skill one must first have a strong desire to do so; they would never force someone to learn from them.

The town was alive with construction activity as thatched-roof dwellings were torn down to make way for larger Western-style dwellings with galvanized roofs, wooden-shuttered windows, cement floors, and frame beds. New skills were in demand. The busiest worker in town was the carpenter, who made doors and windows and guided the framing of a house. He used new tools: a level, a plane, and an L-square. These buildings were angular and symmetrical. A mason mixed cement to lay over previously dirt floors. Shops were springing up selling cigarettes, sugar, cokes, bouillon cubes, salt, matches, and trinkets. Other shops specialized in selling kerosene or rum. There were two tailors in the town with Singer sewing machines. These workers and shops demand cash for their services and goods—no bartering in kind, no exchange of labor.

Talking matter had also noticeably changed. Previously, courts higher than the town chief's court were only an abstraction. People were aware of them, but because of the town's isolation and the lack of cash to meet court costs, the higher courts were not being utilized. The road and cash economy began to change all that. The town chief's and elder's decisions were no longer final. Social control may break down as more and more townspeople no longer feel bound by the dictates of the local court structure. On the other hand, the paramount chief may render a decision, but he is under no obligation to restore order and harmony. The higher courts, due to the Western system under which they operate, give automatic advantage to the litigant who is literate, speaks English, and has plenty of cash. The residents of Gbarngasuakwelle having little or none of these attributes consistently lost court battles with outsiders, including Mandingos. Thus tension between the town world and the *Kwii* world was high.

If the changes that adults are experiencing are great they are nothing compared to the changes in the lives of children. Adults change because it is forced on them. They enter the cash economy primarily because they must pay a government-imposed hut tax. The maneuverings of outsiders force them to go to higher courts to redress their wrongs. They are forced to work on the roads. They are forced to feed, and pay off every government representative who enters their town from a private in the army to the County Commissioner to the paramount chief's messenger. Children, on the other hand, not only feel the pressure to change but are much more open to the inducements of fancy clothes, cassettes, soda pop, and so on.

The next section on play elaborates on these changes in the lives of children.

CHANGES IN PLAY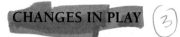

Several new playforms found their way into the town while I was there. The children of Gbarngasuakwelle made two discoveries which, overnight, revolutionized their play practices. These were the wheel and the ball. The wheel came in many manifestations. It may have been on a small car made out of wires or carved out of wood. It may have been an old tire propelled by two sticks, a piece of vine tied in a loop, a bicycle wheel, even a broken lantern with a round base. During the observation period, wheel rolling was the most frequently observed play activity of boys ages 6 to 18. Even when the wheel was a loop of vine, it symbolized the automobile because boys invariably made engine noises as they rolled their wheels. Wheel rolling as car driving was one example among many of the new types of make-believe play. One of the most interesting scenes I witnessed could be labeled "presidential entourage." President Tolbert rode past the town on many occasions enroute to his ranch. He and his aides traveled at high speed in one or two limousines, preceded and followed by police cars that kept their sirens blasting the entire time. People, especially children, hearing the sirens, would run out to the roadside to watch and wave flowers. One day a group of boys reproduced this spectacle. One boy walked in front of the procession making siren-like noises. Another boy, the oldest and tallest of the group, walked behind in his best impression of "stateliness." He was followed by two boys waving scraps of cloth which symbolized the small national flags always flown from the limousines. Other boys walked behind, also erect and dignified, and along their "route," the remaining boys stood waving flowers and shouting greetings to "President Tolbert."

Make-believe play follows closely on the heels of new social customs. The older school boys erected a flag pole outside the "school" on September 25. From that day on the children would "pledge allegiance" to the flag[4] as it was raised every morning before filing inside. On September 29, I witnessed two boys make a miniature flag pole out of bamboo, cut a scrap of cloth into a rectangle, attach it to the pole with string, and then run it up and down the pole, saluting and mumbling something that approximated the pledge of allegiance.

As new forms are introduced, older ones seem quick to disappear. I saw relatively little *Nee-pele* of complex adult skills such as weaving and blacksmithing. Informants, when questioned about *Nee-pele*, would describe various forms in the past tense, indicating that long before, say, leatherworking, ceased to be practiced, children will have given up imitating it in their play.

Changes in hunting are reflected in hunting play (*Sua-kpé pele*). Gun and dog-hunting began to predominate and the various forms of group hunting and bow-and-arrow hunting were waning. Thus *Sua-pele* and *Boloŋ* were disappearing from the play repertoire of young boys, only to be replaced by play centering on the slingshot (actual) and the gun (modeled). Trapping was also waning mainly because young boys and men find gun hunting more exciting. *Gbliŋ Gbe*, the boys' secret society, where initiates were taught medicines to lure animals into traps, was no longer active. Older men started to complain that their sons did not seem interested in learning to trap, preferring instead to go to school.

The play of very young children (i.e., under age 7) seemed to be fairly stable. They continued to imitate their parents and spend a great deal of time in *Loo-pele*, or hiding play, and other traditional games. Slightly older children, however, were going to school and this has had an effect on their play behavior. For example, a modern analogue of *Tiaŋ-kai-sii* is a game in which two boys take turns writing numerals in the sand, at rapid speed, with their fingers. One boy writes "1," the other boy erases it and writes "2," the first boy erases the "2" and writes "3," and so on. This is an example of new forms of drawing play (*Peliŋ-pele*). Schoolchildren were much more likely than their same-age counterparts not attending school to draw pictures or write letters or words in the sand.

Still older boys were turning to imported games. There was one "Ludo" (an English board game with dice) and one "checkers" game in town, and these were both constantly in use by a shifting group of boys from ages 13 to 18. Card games were also catching on rapidly, having been introduced by the schoolteacher and a missionary man living in the village. These foreign games seemed to compete directly with *Bambé*, *Kwatinaŋ*, *Gbaŋ*, "old man spider," and *Malaŋ*, as participation in the traditional games had fallen off sharply in recent times. The case of *Malaŋ* is quite interesting. As I pointed out (Chapter 6), boys learn *Malaŋ* from older men, primarily because these men own the game board and have stored in memory the various strategies for successful play; the Ludo and checkerboards, on the other hand, were owned by young men (both younger than 25). Thus, these games not only represented new playforms but also made boys less dependent on older men and, perhaps, less respectful of them as well. This is only a small instance of a transfer of the authority base from the town's elders to young men who were partially literate and, more important, had lived at least part of their lives outside the town in more Westernized settings.

I have never heard adults more critical of children's behavior than when they were playing ball. Part of the reason was that the adults resented the change represented by the ball games but also because the ball, careening on its course, often struck people and houses. Outside town a soccer field had been laid out, but the goal at one end was about 25 feet off center. The reason for this asymmetry was that directly behind the place where the goal should be was an unfinished house, and the owner of the house complained that the ball too often landed on his new iron roof; hence the goal was shifted. In town, boys kicked around large gourds, cans, and, if any were available, small rubber balls about 18 centimeters in diameter. They had developed a number of games derived from soccer. In one of these, a boy who is "it" trys to kick the ball at anyone from a group of boys who are running around him and trying to avoid being hit. If a boy is hit, he becomes "it" and kicks the ball until he hits someone. Another game was played between two houses. With one or two boys on a side, the teams take turns trying to kick the ball between the houses while the other team tries to block it. Next to wheel rolling, ball games constituted the most frequently observed play activity of boys.

Ball play divided the young from old in the sense that old people had never played, nor were they ever likely to play, with balls. It also divided schoolchildren from those who did not attend school. The soccer field and the one regulation-size ball belonged to the school.[4] Soccer must also be played on a relatively flat surface, which means on the field or in town, and it must be played during daylight. Children who do not attend school spend all day on the farm, where a flat playing surface is impossible to find, so they do not have any opportunity to engage in ball play. I found evidence of a growing gap between the play behavior of children in school compared to that of children not attending school.

The ball and wheel seemed to be connected to larger worlds. Soccer was the national sport of Liberia; all the public schools had soccer teams and the ability to play the game, understand the rules, and so forth seemed to go hand in hand with becoming a student and learning to read, write, and do arithmetic. Significantly, there were no games that involved throwing or batting balls—only kicking. Similarly, wheel rolling was tied to the automobile, which not only represented a powerful and expensive symbol but also connoted the excitement of a trip to the capital city, Monrovia. I introduced the American game of Frisbee into the town to see how a new playform, not buttressed by elaborate symbolism, would be received. Women used plastic buckets with circular lids to carry around their possessions. The buckets wore out before the lids, so there were a fair number of these lids to be found lying around. The lid approximated a Frisbee in shape and size so, on four successive evenings, I used one of them to teach four boys (ages 10 to 13) how to toss a Frisbee. Then, for 2 weeks, my assistant and I monitored children's play for evidence of the game. As my demonstration attracted a substantial audience each time, I believed that the idea was widely diffused. What we found was that for 4 days after the demonstration, there was sporadic Frisbee tossing, primarily by the boys I had taught, but after that we found no sign of it.

No area of play had remained untouched by outside influence, but dancing and musical instruments probably have continued unaltered. The main reason for this is that the traditional forms of music were not so different from Western models that they could not accommodate changes easily. This was especially true of dance steps. Teenagers, however, began to flock to dance to music emanating from a record player as well as to the bands of roving musicians. Clorox bottles filled with seeds were increasingly employed as percussion accompaniment in the songs and dances of young girls. Another new instrument was the guitar, called "gita." A young man brought an example of the Sudanic guitar into the town from Guinea. This instrument has a body made from a large hollow gourd. There is no neck per se and no frets; rather, strips of bamboo are attached to the underside of the gourd and, arching upward, hold the steel strings in suspension to the top of the gourd. The six strings are of uniform thickness but vary in length up to 45 centimeters. The gourd is held in the lap and with both hands resting on either side of the instrument; the player plucks the strings, three with the fingers of his left hand, three with the fingers of his right hand. When the young man played, he was accompanied by a friend on the *Kone*. They played only for the evening dancing and not for ceremonial occasions. Children played a one-stringed steel guitar made from a tin can, a bent sapling, and a steel wire. They plucked at the string with a twig. This "can guitar" was becoming increasingly common but was played only solo and not in accompaniment to singing or dancing. Boys, continued, however, to express their musical abilities through drumming, even beating out rhythms on their textbooks with pencils.

The second of three song types identified (Chapter 7)—long, totally improvised songs—is completely open to new themes. The many songs of this type I recorded all made at least some mention of recently introduced artifacts.

Changes in storytelling and *Koloŋ* were harder to judge. Foreign elements did not seem to have crept into the stories to any appreciable degree. Traditional stories were told in school at the request of the teacher (he is Kpelle). But schoolboys did not tell stories in the evening—which is the normal storytelling time, rather, they read their textbooks and did homework.

Adult play, like adult work, changed less than children's play. Men and women gathered whenever possible for conversation, joking, and gossip. They continued to participate in dancing and music, especially in connection with farmwork. The men played *Malaŋ* and, despite prohibition by the government, gambled at *Gbaŋ*. Nevertheless, my informants perceived that the town was passing through troubled times. The minority group of Mandingos, who were universally distrusted and even hated, was growing. Other outsiders, *Kwii* people, created problems never encountered before. There was, consequently, less *li nee* in the life of the town, and less joy means less play.

Prima facie evidence suggests that there was an overall decline in time allotted to play. In a society in which everyone works on the farm in cooperative work parties, as the number of laborers available declines, the amount of work that falls on to those remaining must increase, assuming no increase in productivity, which was the case here. More time spent in work probably means less time for play. This was in fact happening, Men, young men especially, were leaving the town in increasing numbers to seek wage employment to purchase luxuries. They traveled to Firestone, to Gbarnga, to other nearby towns, and to the President's estate. Their families stayed at home and were expected to make the usual-size rice farm. The men periodically participated in tree felling and burning, but they were lost to the family working unit at other times. Children who were in their working years, especially boys ages 8 to 13, were going to school in increasing numbers; thus, they too, were lost to the working unit for at least two-thirds of the weekly work period. The burden of farming then was falling increasingly on women, young children, and older people. The latter two categories, in particular, appeared to be working more and playing less as time went on.

CHANGES IN LEARNING

Here I would like to catalog briefly the things that children seemed no longer to be learning and might not learn in the future. This includes nearly all skilled work, including blacksmithing, pottery making, leather-work, and cloth weaving. There were some exceptions to this general decline. There had not been as noticeable a decline in girls learning such skills as fishnet weaving, beltbraiding, and bag weaving. Coincidentally, girls were proportionally underrepresented in the public school. In terms of certain skills historically learned by all boys, children still were learning, for example, to weave mats and make traps (although the variety of types was not as great as it used to be). Apprenticeships may have been on the point of disappearing altogether and the the parent–child teaching–learning situation was much declining in evidence.

What had not changed was the learning of such nonskilled work as rice farming, house building, and so on. These tasks, unlike skilled work, were not voluntary; hence children were forced to participate. There had been, however, a sharp shift in the amount of time different groups of children devoted to these nonskilled tasks. Children attending school spent less time working whereas children not attending school spent as much or more time in nonskilled work as before the construction of the road.

To appreciate the new kinds of learning in which children were engaged in requires an examination of the recently introduced public school.

THE NEW SCHOOL

In 1973, a young high school graduate was sent by the government to Gbarngasuakwelle to start a school. He secured permission to hold class in a large new, uninhabited house until a proper building could be erected. The majority of the students started in "primer," a pre-first-grade class, which they stayed in until they mastered sufficient English to handle first grade. Aside from the primer grade, the curriculum, including books and system of instruction, were vintage American. All the students were given biblical first names by the teacher upon matriculation. An important minority of the students had attended school for varying lengths of time outside the town and now returned to attend the local school. These children, all boys, ranged from the first to the seventh grade and a number of them served as assistant teachers.

I found out quickly that there were no typical schooldays, so based on several day's observation spread over 2 months, I created a log of a composite day, which contained all the elements that reoccur with great frequency (Lancy, 1975a). That log illustrates some interesting features of the school.

7:15 A.M. A schoolboy strikes the piece of scrap metal that hangs by the school. This gives off a gong sound that can be heard throughout town. It is the signal to come to school.

8:00 A.M. Children have been gathering in front of the school for the last 20 minutes. An older boy, James forms them into two parallel lines facing the flagpole, tallest at the head of the line to shortest at the tail. James passes among them with a switch telling this one to get in line, that one to stand up straight. There are altogether 69 students, 12 girls, 57 boys; they range in age from 5 to 19; the majority are around 8 to 11. They all wear "uniforms"—bright yellow tops and green bottoms.

8:15 A.M. James blows a whistle and tells the children to "stand at attention." As another older boy raises the flag the children salute and recite: "I pledge allegiance to the flag, of Liberia and to the Republic for which it stands. One nation indivisible, with liberty and justice for all."

8:20 A.M. The children march into the school.

Notice how much time and energy is taken up with ritualized activity. Everyone considered these trappings including, the uniforms, an essential, if not *the* essential, attribute of school. As I have argued (Lancy, 1975b), these rural elementary schools in Liberia were mostly about indoctrination, not education. They were designed to increase villagers' allegiance to the state at the expense of local and tribal affiliations. Children whose parents could not afford school uniforms, were excluded from the school.

8:35 A.M. The teacher arrives and the older boys file into the classroom after him. The first order of business is to put the correct date on the front and rear blackboards. On the left, in the back of the room, are about 30 "primer" students. To their right, are the first-graders, roughly 22 in number. On the right in the front of the room are about 11 second-graders, on the left, we see three fourth-graders and one fifth-grader. The teacher asks for the arithmetic homework from this latter group, and he calls Sammy to the board to work one of the problems, adding $\frac{1}{4} + \frac{1}{8}$. Meanwhile, Monroe and James are working with first- and second-graders, respectively.

For an observer, it is painful to watch. There are so many distractions and the language barrier precludes explanation, so everything is done by rote. The teacher and his assistants make many factual errors in their demonstrations. Nevertheless, aside from the fidgetiness, no one acts as if there is anything wrong with what is going on. Indeed, there is a kind of solemnity about the whole thing that invokes feelings of a religious service.

> 9:45 A.M. The teacher calls the class to attention and he proceeds to read a chapter from a Liberian history book about President Barclay, Liberia's first president.
>
> 10:00 A.M. Recess is declared and the children race into the town. They collect in clusters to talk, fight, and play.
>
> 10:20 A.M. James calls the children back into the classroom, then takes the first- and second-graders outside to do drill. The children carry sticks (as model guns[5]) on their shoulders and practice marching in front of the school—"left, right, left, right," "attention," "about face," "present arms," etc. The teacher works on word recognition with the primer children and the remainder of the older boys work fraction problems.
>
> 11:10 A.M. The children who were marching return to the classroom. Monroe Kollie writes more sentences on the board for the primer class to copy, then calls alternately on first-graders to read from their reading books (*Dick & Jane*). The second-graders now read for James and the older boys read for the teacher. The reading proceeds painfully in all cases. The children have to be threatened before they will attempt to read; they make frequent mistakes and are scolded.

As an outsider, I was struck at first by the dissimilarities between this school and the American model: This one was held in a house, had several grades clustered in one room, had older students as assistant teachers, and so on. But then the similarities emerged and I realized that this classroom, at least superficially, resembled the proverbial "one-room school-house" found in many parts of the United States prior to 1950. The only thing that reminds one that this is not in the United States is the use of Kpelle whenever students were talking among themselves. What was clear was that, regardless of how little "book larnin'" occurred, the children became rapidly socialized to the role of student. They did not question the right of boys only slightly older than themselves (but in higher grades) to order them around, even to beat them. They sat fairly calmly for more than an hour at a time, something they would never do outside the classroom. They suffered embarrassment and humiliation every time they were called on, yet they continue to come back to school. They can not put anything they learn to use outside the classroom yet they do their homework in the evening when other siblings, not attending school, are playing. In the United States there is a long tradition of compulsory education; there is no alternative for a child in terms either of law or tradition but to go to school. These children, however, were not required either by law or by tradition to go to school, so why did they go?

This question has at least three answers, all of which contribute in some measure to motivating a child to attend school. The first reason is quite simple but very important. If a child is not attending school in the morning, he or she is expected to work on the farm, and children seem more than willing to trade the intellectual and emotional labor of the school for the physical labor of the farm. Second, children see schooling as part fulfillment of their desire to become *Kwii*. For students, speaking English, "knowing book," and wearing Western-style uniforms all add to a desirable self-image. This reasoning was especially marked in the older students, and they consciously used the teacher as a model. They visited his home to listen to his tape recorder, to talk to him about his experiences, and so on. When he went to town for visits they surrounded him on his return. In short, he represented everything they were striving for so they willingly subjugated their own will to his. Thus, the students' relationship to their teacher was strikingly similar to the traditional apprenticeship (see Chapter 9). The children, especially the older ones, also see the school as an essential step in becoming *Kwii* (i.e., "Do anything you have to go to school."). In their conversations they talked endlessly about wanting to visit Monrovia or the United States. Their social studies text gives them tantalizing glimpses of the United States, as it was written for American schools. They were gradually learning an equation: school = job = money = travel = luxury items.

A third motivating factor was the attitude of parents. Many parents wanted at least one of their children to attend school because they believed that their *Kwii* children would protect them from exploitation by educated outsiders. They provided the money to purchase uniforms, pens, and pencils and continued feeding and sheltering the child even though he was no longer doing farmwork full time. If the parents did not want a child to attend school, they simply stopped giving the child food until he or she returned to work on the farm. Indeed, Dennis (1972) suggests of the Gbandes that only the laziest, least-promising boys were sent to school; other children, especially girls, were kept at home to work.

From an extended interview, I recorded the following comments concerning the efficacy of schooling: "Right now they [*Kwii* people] are squeezing us, but they won't take our children's chickens. If our children go to school people will be afraid of them and won't abuse them the way they abuse us." But the children should not become so *Kwii* that they turn on their own parents and abuse them (e.g., "You have suffered to educate him now he left you lying down in a dirty place, mosquitoes are sucking you, no food to eat. That boy is enjoying his girlfriend, buying his friends rum, he has forgotten you."). James was a model son in this regard. His father, Nang Kollie, sent him away to school because James was slightly lame and unable to do farmwork very well. Today James lives with his family, works on their farm, and, most important, acts as go-between whenever his father must deal with a *Kwii* person. He defended his father in court against charges that his father had failed to pay the hut tax, for example. The ideal, then, was for each family to have at least one son who had enough education to pass as *Kwii* (i.e., he should be able to speak English, know enough math to buy and sell, and be able to read and write), but not so much education that he would leave the town permanently and no longer be able to protect his family.

Therefore, there are two views of the school. The children who attended it saw it as leading to revolutionary changes in their own lives. They hoped it would lead them from the isolation of Gbarngasuakwelle, from farm labor and from their parents' domination. The adults hold an opposite view. They want educated children to serve as a "perimeter around the town," protecting it from outsiders. In other respects they do not want their children to change; they want them to stay at home,[6] to continue to farm and learn traditional skills, and to remain under their guidance and control. Thus the town was sharply divided over whether to build a permanent school building outside the town. The children, of course, were in favor of it, as was the teacher. The government ordered that one be built; hence, the chief felt compelled to see that it was built, but the majority of the men, even those who were already sending their children to school, were opposed to it and contributed their labor only under the threat of fines if they refused. They saw no reason to continue public schooling indefinitely; only long enough to produce an educated cadre of residents to counter the effects of Mandingos, soldiers, messengers, and commissioners.

THE PUBLIC SCHOOL AND APPRENTICESHIP

It would be fruitful to compare the process of schooling to the traditional apprenticeship (Greenfield & Lave, 1982) because one seems to have supplanted the other. Both are long-term processes. Both involve a designated teacher or master. Both take place in the teacher's domain (locationally) rather than in the student's domain. Both involve the application of verbal abuse and corporal punishment by the teacher (or his surrogates) to wayward students. Both involve the acquisition of some higher status on completion because of the ability to execute special skills (e.g., reading or weaving cloth). Both involve learning some foundation skills, and some applied skills although the proportions are vastly different for the two processes. That is, apprenticeship requires applied knowledge whereas schooling emphasizes basic skills or "foundations." Both may lead to a degree of independence from the routines of rice farming. The apprentice may be able to trade products for farm labor, whereas the schooled individual may be able to trade cash earned from a job for food. The failed apprentice and the failed student, however, will both "return to the farm" (i.e., will have to earn their sustenance from rice farming).

There are, of course, differences between the two processes. In apprenticeship, learning is achieved primarily through observation, imitation, and practice, with some direction by the master (usually only disapproval or approval). To a certain extent, the same kind of copying goes on in the classroom, as well as the same rewards and punishments, but education in school also requires that the student combine what he has learned to solve never-before-encountered problems and to create original ideas and structures. Another difference is that the school is a group affair whereas apprenticeship pairs a master with a single apprentice. The apprentice compares his or her progress to the master's model or to his or her own previous best work, whereas students judge themselves against other students. Hence, the term "failure" takes on a different meaning in the two cases. One can fail to make a knife properly, but, in the classroom, one can fail simply because one has the lowest scores on tests.

In school, all students were learning the "same things" and, after being schooled, all students take on a new status as *Kwii*. In this aspect, the school in Gbarngasuakwelle more closely resembled initiation into *Poro* or *Sande* than apprenticeship. In fact, one can argue that both initiation and apprenticeship were being supplanted by the school. Both public school and *Poro/Sande* lead the child into universalistic associations because both institutions transcend the boundaries of town and tribe. But the chief difference that makes the school the most profound change agent of the many introduced into Gbarngasuakwelle is the tendency of the school to lead children to expect, even to seek out, change in their own lives and in the town. It leads them to reject the traditions of their fathers, the work and the play that characterize their culture. Apprenticeship and initiation lead the child in conservative directions. The skilled worker resists change because it endangers his or her livelihood. The *Poro* and *Sande* societies continually reinforce the religious and political status quo because their power to enforce social control stems from deep-seated traditions, special knowledge, and medicines which *Zò-na* and other powerful figures control.

The school serves numerous functions in the eyes of those who created it and those who try to make it work in Gbarngasuakwelle. There are serious questions as to whether the children of the town will actually acquire an "education" in the Western sense. What can not be questioned, however, is the success of the school, in less than a year, in *indoctrinating* students to the benefits of *Kwii*ness.

THE *KWII* WAY IS A DEAD-END STREET

As the epigram that opened this chapter suggests, the number of individuals in the third world who complete a course of study and end up in well-paying jobs is a minuscule fraction of the millions who start out in primary school with high hopes (see also Serpell, 1993). This observation is based on global analysis of the present state of childhood education and development—especially in the third world. LeVine and White (1986) identify several reasons why public schooling is not working, not the least of which is its prohibitive cost. Given what we know about the facilitative effects of such middle-class child-rearing routines as the bedtime story, when these routines are missing the school must somehow find substitutes,[7] and these will inevitably drive up the cost. Thus, schools in the third world need to spend much more on public schooling than do the industrialized countries to achieve comparable results.

With rare exceptions (Jahoda, 1983; Price-Williams, Gordon, & Ramirez, 1969), the routines that function well to transmit the indigenous culture do not work very well in preparing children to succeed in school (Phillips, 1983). Further, such school readiness and support routines as the bedtime story are not easily acquired by parents who, themselves, have never been schooled.[8] Evidence in the industrialized world indicates a close relationship between children's academic success and their mother's level of education. But, the Kpelle, in common with other traditional societies (e.g., Pomponio & Lancy, 1986) discourage girls from going to school. Even when the Kpelle desire a son to attend school, they look upon it with the same attitude they hold toward helping him become a competent Kpelle: "It's up to the child." Parents in other societies (Lareau, 1989;

Levin, 1990) in which children gain little benefit from their schooling hold similar attitudes.

Sutton-Smith (1977) points out the inherent limitation in the tendency to rely upon sibling caretakers in terms of school readiness: "Maximal personal and social development of infants is produced by the mother (or caretaker) who interacts with them in a variety of stimulating and playful ways. Unfortunately the intelligence to do this with ever more exciting contingencies is simply not present in child caretakers. It is difficult enough to impart these ideas of infant stimulation even to mothers" (p. 184). But, perhaps, this "gap" can be closed by changing the instruction in school to better allow the child to utilize his knowledge of his own culture?

For example, Gerdes's (1988) solution to the problem of the "educational failure of many children from third world countries and from ethnic minority communities in industrialized countries ... [would be] to (*multi*)*culturalise* the school curriculum ... [subjects should] be 'imbedded' into the cultural environment of the pupils" (p. 35). As my review (Lancy, 1994a, 1994b) shows, attempts to do this actually have not met with great success. First, children seem quickly to abandon traditional playforms on which the multicultural curriculum might be expected to build. deMarrais, Nelson, and Baker (1992) studied Yup'ik Eskimo girls' "storyknife" drawing/storytelling. These are clearly a rich resource in teaching girls about their culture. But, alas, "We thought that our work could inform teachers who work with Yup'ik Eskimo children, but now found that with so few children engaged in this activity, this strategy may no longer be appropriate" (p. 121).

We encountered a second problem in our work with the Ministry of Education in Papua New Guinea. Parents were supportive of the public schools insofar as they saw their children moving inexorably into the *Kwii* (or in Papua New Guinea *Whitepela*) world. Any deviation from that path, which might be suggested in the incorporation of elements from the village curriculum, was summarily opposed (Pomponio & Lancy, 1986). Third, we really are talking about rocket science. The relaxed laissez-faire quality of enculturation in the village is simply incompatible with the enormous volume of information children must master in school in a short period. In the developed nations, children as young as 6 can readily be identified as falling so far behind in acquiring knowledge as to be unlikely to catch up. By contrast, children in Gbarngasuakwelle can take years to master the simple arithmetic involved in buying and selling. Two separate, large-scale studies (Cole et al., 1971; Lancy, 1983) found that Kpelle students and their Papua New Guinean counterparts spend at least

4 years in school before they reliably begin to use more efficient information-processing strategies (e.g., Piaget's concrete operations). Further, research conducted by economists in rural Liberia in the late 1960s revealed that tribal peoples, like the Kpelle, would need at least a tenth-grade education before schooling paid any monetary benefits (John Gay, personal communication, September 23, 1994).

Not surprisingly, then, the majority who drop out along the way have not achieved a sufficient level of mastery of these new skills, such as literacy, to continue using and developing them once they leave school (Serpell, 1993). Moreover, they are given relatively little incentive to do so in the daily round of village life. Government planners push universal primary schooling in the hope that "school leavers" will bring modern ideas of health, sanitation, finance, and agriculture to their natal society. Such rarely happens. Indeed, school leavers who attempt to bring change to the village are called *frisky* in Liberia and *bikhet*[9] in Papua New Guinea (Pomponio & Lancy, 1986). It is significant that Kpelle parents want at least some children to become *Kwii*, so they do not have to become *Kwii* themselves.

None of this would be so discouraging if there were not a further serious problem built into this precipitate rush down the *Kwii* road. Nearly 50 years ago Leighton and Kluckhohn (1948) first documented the insidious effect of Western schooling on the maintenance of culture as information (see Chapter 2). As one of their student informants lamented: "I do not know any sings because I am in school studying things. I never seen *Yebichai* yet" (p. 69). Even though Gbarngasuakwelle's introduction to the *Kwii* road is recent, my informants and I were already able to detect the abandonment of cultural routines that are essential in transmitting Kpelle culture to the next generation. The rub is that the very hands-off, autotelic quality of these routines dooms them to extinction. That is, as I have illustrated throughout this book, the Kpelle traditional educational system works beautifully without anyone being in charge, without schedules, without parental anxiety. There is no board of education to which to complain, no teachers to "in-service," no superintendent to fire, no curriculum to be revised, no new technology to purchase. No one is in charge; hence, no single adult feels the responsibility to, say, organize, storytelling tournaments to keep the *Meni-pele* genre alive.

Is there an alternative road to travel? I do not think so, but the loss of culture can at least be slowed by the elimination of universal primary schooling—one of the worst ideas foisted on the third world by well-meaning but short-sighted bureaucrats from the developed nations. While with the Ministry of Education in Papua New Guinea, I recommended (Lancy, 1979) that the government continue funding the primary schools at the same or a higher level but cut enrollments by 33–50% and let the villagers themselves decide who should go to school and who should stay at home to learn the culture. However, because foreign aid is contingent upon third world nations paying at least lip service to a litany of goals such as universal primary education, the country was unable to do this. We did find, however, that villagers had taken matters into their own hands and enrollment in village primary schools started to drop off dramatically (Pomponio & Lancy, 1986).

The Kpelle and the people of Gbarngasuakwelle and of Liberia are now facing a terrible future. The *Kwii* road has been a dead end, the investment in public schooling did not pay off in terms of a dramatically transformed economy of modernized agriculture and industry—it just made more people aware of how "poor" they were, of how many wondrous things they lacked the cash to purchase. On the other hand, unchecked population growth has meant that the traditional way of life is also no longer viable. The bush is being eaten, its plant and animal resources depleted. Fallow periods are growing shorter and yields declining—a vicious circle. Ultimately, thin, fragile tropical soils are completely depleted. The result is the unending, brutal civil war that has engulfed Liberia and that threatens to destroy most of Africa (see also Johnston & Low, 1995, for a parallel horror story from Guatemala).

I write these words shortly after writing a lengthy essay on the state of the world's children (Lancy, 1995). It is a grim picture. The only hope lies in a reversal of our national and international myopia regarding contraception. Sensitive and open-minded research by ecologial anthropologists in recent years has shown that the kind of subsistence practices followed by slash-and-burn horticulturalists such as the Kpelle, far from being inefficient, are wonderfully adapted to the local ecology. The Kpelle do not need the Green Revolution. Village-based societies such as Gbarngasuakwelle are also remarkably self-sufficient in terms of producing nonfood necessities—housing, crockery, clothing, and tools. They do not need to depend on expensive, energy and resource-wasteful manufactured items. In short, the village-based subsistence economy may well represent an optimal adaptive strategy—one that can endure indefinitely. But villagers do need some form of cheap, reliable contraception because overpopulation destroys this delicate balance.

As this book has shown, the long-term viability of the village economy and way of life is also supported by a stock-in-trade of cultural routines that work effectively to prepare children to carry on these traditons and skills. As discussed in Chapter 2, Spencer in 1899 called attention to the powerful relationship between the kinds of experiences a society provides its children and the kinds of social, intellectual, and technical competencies mastered by adults. This relationship is fundamentally a conservative one; children learn what they see around them. Societies depend on this inherent desire for children to copy their elders and on the wonderful ability of the young of our species to observe, imitate, and self-correct. In a village such as Gbarngasuakwelle, much of human life is conducted in the open and children are encouraged to stick around and watch. Since time immemorial, games have been played, dances danced, and songs sung, and, according to virtually every authority, all these also contribute, conveniently, to the child's education. Societies create tasks and tools in miniature, sized to the frame and skill of the growing child. Children welcome opportunities to participate while their labor is appreciated by the household. For adolescents, societies organize rites of passage in which critical cultural values are imparted and apprenticeships during which complex and critical skills are conveyed. I have called all these activities and situations cultural routines for children's development and have attempted to demonstrate their importance in sustaining an entire way of life.

Notes

CHAPTER 1

1. This is an important milestone in many societies. For the Kipsigis, the child is said to have sense or *ng'om* when not only can they take care of themselves, but they can undertake certain routine chores (e.g., watering the cows and sweeping the house) without supervision (Super & Harkness, 1986).

2. I am grateful to John Singleton, whose course in education and anthropology and chairmanship of my dissertation, contributed much to the methodology described here.

3. Another ethnographer who used Ricks's able services was Bledsoe (1980). She says: "Thanks to his patience, humor and tact, even normally reticent women talk readily to him" (p. 5). High praise, indeed!

4. A. A. Kulah (1973), who studied Kpelle children's acquisition of proverbs, noted that his principal informants seemed well aware of the function of a tape recorder: "How can you lie when this witch [the tape recorder] here will expose you?" (p. 40).

5. I took two photos of each child, one of which I gave to the child. This single gesture earned me a high level of cooperation from the town as a whole and especially from my principal subjects.

CHAPTER 2

1. Another trade-off relates to the relative prevalence of girls versus boys. In many parts of the world, males are preferred and parents exert subtle influences that skew child survival to favor males (e.g., Das Gupta, 1987). However, Cronk (1993) has published an important study based on research with the Mukogodo of Tanzania. For reasons I do not have space to discuss, women have an easier time marrying than men do and, hence, are more likely to have children. Athough mothers *claim* to prefer boys, their behavior shows otherwise. Daughters are breast-fed longer than sons, boys are malnourished, and their festering sores are more likely to be neglected. Consequently, the sex ratio, 50–50 at birth, shifts to 60–40 in favor of girls by age 5.

2. This statement applies only to the !Kung as hunters and gatherers (Draper, 1976). In a remarkable study, Draper and Cashdan (1988) showed that as the !Kung were forced to become sedentary agriculturists, their approach to child rearing more closely resembled the "child-supported" model (Figure 2.1). There was less parent—child interaction and more sibling caretaking, and children were expected to make an economic contribution to the household from an early age.

3. "The Sebei say that a man who dies without children is forgotten; his name is thrown away; his spirit is dead. . . . a barren wife is scorned and shamed, for reproduction is seen as her prime purpose" (Goldschmidt, 1976, p. 243).

4. When we read in the popular press about Bangladeshi parents selling their boys to serve as camel jockeys in the Persian Gulf (McCarron, 1993), or about 19 children living in filth and squalor in a Chicago tenement, despite a household income of $4,000 a month (Biema, 1994), we should examine the cultural traditions that bring this about. In these cases a cash income may be both essential to survival and otherwise unobtainable. In the African American ghettos of Chicago, the only "legitimate" source of income for many women may be Aid to Families with Dependent Children. Earning this income is contingent upon having offspring who survive. That is the only requirement. Given the high murder rate in Chicago, is it any wonder that these parents lean toward the R strategy (Harris, 1989). The children were born of four sisters who, by jointly raising their children, are "hedging their bets"; if one sister is unlucky in the survival rate of her offspring, she has the consolation that her genes are also carried by her nieces and nephews, whose survival she has contributed to.

5. My colleague John Gay, whose association with the Kpelle goes back more than 30 years, took me to task for this sweeping generalization. He wrote: "You very much overstate the case on rules for marriage . . . we all know there are many marital patterns among the Kpelle . . ." (personal communication, September 23, 1994). Point taken. Marriage patterns are subject to considerable variation, as are the routines for child rearing. But I do think my general point still holds.

6. In her initial review, editor Sara Harkness (November 18, 1994) noted that although many "neo"-Vygotskians assume that parents are conscious teachers, Vygotsky, himself, never made that claim.

7. To the extent that Freud's and Piaget's theories were framed by the bourgeois society of Western Europe, Vygotsky was also clearly determined to fashion a version of developmental psychology more compatible with the communist society of Soviet Russia.

8. Consider the raging debate in contemporary U.S. society concerning the teaching of values–socialization. The majority still think of this as the responsibility of family, church, and community, whereas the school should be responsible for education–enculturation.

9. Roy D'Andrade (1984) has continued to develop many of these ideas. He has coined the term "cultural meaning systems."

> Analytically, cultural meaning systems can be treated as a very large diversified pool of knowledge, or partially shared clusters of norms, or as intersubjectively shared symbolically created realities. On the individual level, however, the actual meanings and messages that people learn, encounter, and produce are typically not divided into separate classes of items that can be labeled knowledge, norm, or reality, but rather form multifunctional complexes of constructs, organized in interlocking hierarchical structures, which are simultaneously constructive, representative, evocative, and directive. (p. 116)

10. Think of our system of education as a gigantic warehouse of useful routines—textbooks, times tables, tape players, blackboards, lessons, curricula, computer programs, atlases—for enculturating the next generation.

11. Pfeiffer (1982) theorizes about cave paintings as information storage devices: "If their art is any indication, the people of the upper Paleolithic . . . confronted with an increasingly complex way of life and pile up of information . . . were engaged in the first large-scale effort to organize knowledge for readier long term retention and recall" (p. 215). Johnson's (1989) analysis of footprint patterns shows that the majority of visitors to prehistoric caves were children or adolescents. "My suggestion is that children visiting the Pyrenees caves were age cohorts organized into initiation groups to experience what we term *initiation* and *rite of passage*" (p. 246).

12. The Latin term *ludus* nominally means "game," but, to the Romans, it also connoted imitation of adults and school. "Learning was a game, *ludus*, because children merely went through the motions: they only imitated action" (Dupont, 1992, p. 226).

13. My colleague John Gay writes from Lesotho: "Basotho children are just like the Ngoni in their desire to get into the countryside to herd animals. But, it is changing, as people realize that being a herdboy is a dead-end occupation" (personal communication, September 23, 1994).

14. Ethnographers often make implicit use of this notion—I did—in conducting what amounts to cultural stratigraphy. That is, we consciously seek out older, articulate individuals to observe and learn about the old ways. We are drawn, as well, to "culture brokers," individuals who seem to have one foot in the present and one foot in the future.

15. Lest I be accused of ethnocentrism, here is a juicy example from our own society. Valsiner (1989b, pp. 181–182) has a wonderful discussion of how the U.S. medical establishment, having decided that many children's problems stemmed from "spoiling" them, launched a disinformation campaign against cradles. Very successful, this campaign ended what had been for centuries an extremely effective cultural routine for comforting babies.

CHAPTER 3

1. While in the Moluccas in 1858, Alfred Russel Wallace—Darwin's theoretical rival—had a malarial attack and wrote in his diary, "during one of these fits, while again considering the problem of the origin of the species, . . . there suddenly flashed upon me the idea of the *survival of the fittest* . . ." (Milner, 1991, p. 53). I was just plain sick.

CHAPTER 4

1. The student of learning and education in societies in which children are expected to learn by observation, can have a difficult time; for example, "I felt the absence of formal teaching quite trying . . . and not very helpful to my endeavors to familiarize myself with the culture" (Nicolaisen, 1988, p. 206; see also Henze, 1992).

2. During Kulah's (1973) study of proverb learning among the Kpelle, mentioned in Chapter 1, the old men he interviewed referred to him as "new palm oil in an old gourd" (p. 37) meaning that although young (he was 27), he demonstrated proper deference, including the correct speech forms, in addressing these older men.

3. These kitchens are built exactly like those in the cylindrical house only on a smaller scale. The main purpose in having a separate kitchen is to mitigate against the danger of fire.

CHAPTER 5

1. For a comparable study done in the Cameroons, see Nsamenang and Lamb (1994).

2. An illustrative example comes from Whiting and Edwards's (1988) analysis, namely, the tendency for mainstream parents to travel with toys, books, and games to ensure that their offspring's minds will be active during every waking moment.

3. As sharp as the contrast is between American middle-class and Kpelle enculturation practices, an equally instructive contrast can be drawn between our own practices and those of the members of the middle class in the Far East, whose investment in the academic preparedness of their offspring is, quite evidently, greater than our own. LeVine and White (1986) describe a cultural routine found in Japan (see also Lebra, 1994):

The home-study desk bought by most parents for their smaller children symbolizes the hovering care and intensity of the mother's involvement: all models have a high front and half-sides, cutting out distractions and enclosing the workspace in womb-like protection. There is a built-in study light, shelves, a clock, electric pencil sharpener and built-in calculator. The most popular recent model included a push button connecting to a buzzer in the kitchen to summon mother for help or for a snack. (p. 123)

4. This relationship, in culture, between the amount of information a member needs to acquire to become competent and the length of the period of dependency parallels the relationship in biology. That is, the argument most commonly made (Konner, 1990) to explain why human (and other great ape) infants remain helpless for so long is that it takes the mother a long time to teach her offspring all the things an omnivorous and opportunistic species needs to know to make a living. So, too, we would expect that the society would lengthen the period of dependency ("You're not old enough for that!") to match the time it took an untalented child to master the minimal requirements for adult citizenship. In American society, this lengthening of the period of immaturity can be tracked historically (consider drinking age, school-leaving age, child labor statutes) as can the growth in the knowledge base considered prerequisite to employment, parenthood, economic independence, and community participation.

5. The antiquity of these practices might surprise some. In Athens during the classic period, "infants and toddlers were catered to through special equipment, feeding bottles, potty stools, cradles, perhaps walkers" (Golden, 1990, p. 17).

6. According to several recent studies (reviewed in Konner, 1990), frequent nursing is associated with elevated levels of prolactin, which in turn reduces the level of hormones implicated in conception. Hence, nursing mothers are less likely to get pregnant.

7. Mother–child play may be absent as well. Harkness and Super (1986) report for the Kipsigis, an East African Nilotic group, that "in 2-hour recordings of child language at home in naturally occurring situations for a sample of 21 children, there are no instances of mothers playing with their children" (p. 102).

8. A comparison of mother–child interaction among West African immigrant women in Paris with their French counterparts shows similar, striking differences (Rabain-Jamin, 1994). For example, "Immigrant African mothers do not usually talk to their children during child care or diapering, which, in contrast, are rich exchange periods for French and American mothers" (p. 156).

9. A fair proportion of the earliest printed books were advice manuals for parents and these focused largely on enculturation for good manners—proper behavior for polite society (Rickert, 1966).

10. The unhurried nature of child development coupled with the existence of multiple caretakers significantly lightens the caretaking responsibilities of parents

in nonindustrialized societies. When families from such communities migrate to cities, this situation dramatically changes. The expectation of "society" that parents will socialize their children for school, keep them dressed "properly," and monitor their schoolwork, all without the aid of other caretakers, is often too much to bear. Child abuse/abandonment rates are extremely high in such urban migrant communities, even among Pacific Islanders who are noted—in the traditional societies—for indulging and cherishing their young children (Boyden, 1991).

11. Not all societies subscribe to the mother-ground concept. In the Marquesas, parents do not want kids "hanging around." They chase them away and are unconcerned about children's exposure to manifest dangers: the sea, sharp rocks, broken glass, and knives (Martini, 1994). Indeed, the Marquesas are noteworthy also in the extreme autonomy of the mixed-age play group in which children are quite clearly "raised" by other children, as is the case with urban street children (Boyden, 1991; see also Zukow, 1989).

12. The series coeditor Sara Harkness queried here: "You offer a somewhat disturbing commentary on destructiveness in relation to both toys and animals but do not explain. Can you suggest why?" It is puzzling. I have observed children acting in a "cruel" manner to animals in Liberia and, extensively, in Papua New Guinea. Dogs are routinely stoned or beaten with sticks if foolish enough to come in range. Bateson and Mead (1942) show a photographic sequence of a toddler "playing with" a tiny bird tethered on a string. In 1968, in Sinyéé village, I purchased a mongoose from its tormentors and it became my pet, nestling happily in my pocket or cuff. This was treated as yet another example of my weird, not to say crazy, behavior. Far from reprimanding children for damaging animals or property, parents tolerate considerable physical abuse from their under-4-year-olds directed at their own persons. I can only speculate that in the societies I have observed, they value property less than we do, are less sentimental about animals than we are, and are less sanguine about the prospects for socializing young children—who are considered to be rather wild and untamable before a certain age.

13. The widespread reporting of make-believe play in contemporary societies is also true of the historical record. An Egyptian mastaba from the tomb of Mereruka in Saqquara from ca. 2300 B.C. depicts boys playing at war. Some boys are dressed as soldiers, one has his hands bound—a captive. In a lower panel, girls have formed a living merry-go-round and the inscription refers to their activity as "pressing the grapes." "Starting from about five years of age, children began to prepare themselves, through play, for adult work" (Strouhal, 1990, p. 190).

CHAPTER 6

1. On a historical note, Moore and Roberts were at Yale and Cornell, respectively, at the time they first broached these ideas. Both were to move to the

University of Pittsburgh somewhat later, where they were to remain. Despite this propinquity and their obvious common interest, the only time they ever collabo- rated, to my knowledge, was in service on my dissertation committee in advising me on the research reported in this volume.

2. I did not pursue the "origins" of Kpelle playforms, nor was I able to ex- amine the role of games in earlier periods of Kpelle history. Nevertheless, it is in- teresting to speculate on whether any games such as *Pili* or *Malaŋ* may have served as a proxy for warfare. This use of games and other contests is not uncommon, even among so-called simple societies. Vennum (1994), for example, calls lacrosse the "little brother of war," as it *was* used in dispute settlement by northeastern (North American) tribes. *Pili* would also qualify for Schwartzman's (1978) "social formaldehyde" (p. 328) theory of play—that playforms preserve patterns of think- ing and behaving that no longer operate in the culture proper.

3. One of the most important documents in the history of civilization is a cuneiform tablet from Ur that has been characterized as a "Farmer's Almanac" (Kramer, 1963). It provides a manual for the prospective grain farmer of all the steps in the process from field preparation to winnowing. What makes this docu- ment so significant is that the didactic manual is prefaced by the phrase "In days of yore, a farmer instructed his son . . . " suggesting that the author knew he was experiencing a watershed in the transition from preliterate to literate society and from informal to more formal means of enculturation (see also Chapter 10, this volume). A fascinating parallel occurred on April 2, 1995. Driving to the office— where I was to spend the day revising this chapter—my wife was complaining about her lack of confidence in the outcome of the sweet pea seeds she had plant- ed the day before. Joyce grew up on a farm and sweet peas were one of the inau- gural plants in the annual vegetable garden. But her parents never explained or verbalized any of the hundreds of rules of thumb regarding the planting and nur- turance of their crops. Because she withdrew from farm labor to attend school be- fore these routines had been committed to memory through sheer practice, Joyce's mental schema for vegetables is spotty at best. Yesterday at the Seed and Feed store, she was about to purchase a packet of sweet pea seeds—conveniently with directions printed on the reverse—but allowed the clerk to talk her into buying a "much better" variety that was only available in bulk (i.e., no directions).

4. Another "play" secret society is discussed in the next chapter.

5. I learned it from adult informants.

6. Strategic skills are those intellectual and personal qualities that are re- quired for success at games of strategy (Roberts & Sutton-Smith, 1962).

7. Athletic contests—wrestling is prevalent in parts of West Africa—tend to occur when males are organized into age–grade ranks and where a warrior ethos is still present (Ottenberg, 1989). We would also expect to see much more play in-

volving weapons and stalking prey in societies that depended on young males' hunting and fishing proficiency (e.g., the Ijaw—Leis, 1972; and the !Kung—Lee, 1979).

8. Kpelle children have the "luxury" of same-age play groups (see also Nydegger & Nydegger, 1963, on the Tarong). In societies in which villages or hamlets are much smaller than Gbarngasuakwelle, playgroups will, of necessity, span a wider age range. This was the case in the six societies I studied in Papua New Guinea. An interesting corollary is that none of the games in these societies is nearly as complex as many of the Kpelle games because of the ceiling effect imposed by having players as young as four in these mixed-age groups (Lancy, 1984).

9. The data are lacking that would enable a similar study of other game sets and some sets might be incomplete owing to the extinction of many traditional games.

10. Schwartzman (1978) identifies a major divide in the literature on this point: "Games . . . are treated as if they are a *context* only for the *expression* (and not the generation) of specific cognitive skills" (pp. 281–282). Piaget (1951) is the principal author of the expression view, whereas Jerome Bruner (1975) has been one of the principal authors of the generation view. Although I tend to side with the latter, the data reported here are, unfortunately, inadequate as a means to resolve this debate.

CHAPTER 7

1. Laziness in Africa is often "ridicule[d] through speech and song" (Ottenberg, 1989, p. 119). The following song, collected by Ocitti (1973) from the East African Acholi, is a wonderful example:

> The mother of this girl
> Dies on the way to the well.
> On the grinding stone.
> In the fields picking vegetables.
> In the bush collecting firewood.
> As if she has no children.
> A hopeless daughter she has
> A daughter who has no manners,
> Who is beautiful for nothing.
> The mother of this girl,
> Suffers all day long.
> As if she has not delivered. (p. 11)

2. Throughout the rather extensive research on stories I was unable to find girls or women who would willingly tell stories. Therefore, I assumed that females do not tell stories. Later I learned that Judy Gay had collected many stories from

women in other Kpelle towns. Her collection is now housed in the Archives of Traditional Music at the University of Indiana. It may be that females in Gbarngasuakwelle do not tell stories or that, because I lacked a female assistant, females were too shy to tell me or my assistant any stories. Unfortunate for supporting this latter position is the fact that females willingly sang songs, told *Koloŋ*, and played games in our presence. On the other hand, Judy Gay's informants all came from the relatively acculturated area around Cuttington College. Hence, the women may have felt less compunction about invading a male domain, especially, in a *Kwii* home. The stories Dr. Gay collected were not, in any event, noticeably different structurally or thematically from those I collected.

3. The procedure for recording and translating stories, songs and *Koloŋ* was as follows:

a. *Tape recording.* All the stories, songs and *Koloŋ* reproduced in this chapter were initially recorded on a cassette tape recorder.

b. *Transcription.* Each recording was played back before a group of three to four informants, always including the person who had originally supplied the story, song, or *Koloŋ*, while my research assistant transcribed them into phonetic Kpelle on paper. The informants would discuss each line or phrase so that an exact transcription could be achieved. This was necessary because at many points in the recordings, especially of songs, the text was garbled or masked by extraneous noises. Phrases would be replayed as many as five times before all informants were satisfied that the transcription was correct.

c. *Literal translation.* Two informants who spoke English worked with my assistant to translate the transcribed Kpelle literally into English.

d. *Meaningful translation.* The literal translations were not always meaningful so my research assistant and I conducted a second transformation. I would read the literal translation and then suggest to my assistant changes that would retain the original meaning but reflect conventional English grammar and usage.

e. *Analysis of meaning.* Even after the final English translation, many phrases and terms remained that required explication (e.g., proverbs, nicknames, and ideophones). These explanations appear in parenthesis throughout the stories, songs, and *Koloŋ* in this chapter.

4. Henries (1966), who has published a major collection of Liberian—especially Kpelle—folklore, claims that "woman palaver" is a dominant theme. These are polygynous societies where jealousy among women seems endemic. Barren women are often the villains of these tales and beautiful women often end up as unfortunate victims.

5. Rather "elementary," we might say, in comparison to the Balinese. But then, having visited Bali and being familiar with the ethnographic literature, I would say that it takes much more "education" to become Balinese than to become Kpelle. Hobart (1988) has studied the educational significance of the Balinese shadow play (*Wayang Kulit*) and operetta (*Arja*).

Children constitute the front rows of any audience, their attention being riveted on the servants who clown around and tell spicy, bawdy jokes. Young children, up to about ten or twelve years old, are drawn to any performance irrespective of the dramatic genre, while small infants sit on their parents' laps for hours at night, sometimes until late into the morning, often lapsing into sleep. As adolescence is reached, in line with the sexual dichotomy which runs through social life and thought, boys frequent the shadow play more and girls the operetta. So the system of morality, together with the history and cosmology represented in the plays, is largely unconsciously adopted, and the molding of the individual to the social norms occurs imperceptibly and indirectly as a pleasurable "by-product" as it were of the cultural routine. (p. 133)

Some of the values represented include proper relations between husbands and wives and a rationale for polygyny. Fundamental moral precepts—"refinement versus coarseness"—are illustrated and parents draw on characters from the theater to use, illustratively, when giving instructive talks to children. Boys do make-believe shadow plays using banana leaves and bamboo rods. Girls do the operettas. "It is in their play-acting that children explore the different dramatic stimuli and the meaning they encapsulate" (p. 138).

CHAPTER 8

1. Aside from the obvious value of the child's labor to the parent, there are two minimal criteria in judging the worth of a parent: their children's manners and their work ethic. Children who are unable or unwilling to work give their parents a bad reputation (Chapter 5).

She is taught to do exactly as her mother does, so that when the mother goes anywhere, she will return home to find the work done. If the mother finds the work improperly done, she . . . abuses the girl . . . , saying: "I hope that you have stomach pains and dysentery." Mothers are concerned that their daughters learn proper housekeeping so that their husbands will not beat them for neglecting their duties, and so it will not be said that they failed to learn proper behavior from their mother. (Goldschmidt, 1976, p. 259)

2. It should be noted that this difference in the degree of "protectiveness" is also motivated by contrasting reproductive strategies (see Chapter 2).

3. Using a camera comes to mind as an example of staged learning from my own enculturation. I watched my father use a single-lens reflex camera (SLR) and we had slide evenings every few months during which he would severely judge his own efforts. At about age 10, I was given a "Brownie" for my birthday. Over time, I graduated to color slides from black-and-white prints and to my own (cheap) SLR. At about 18, I started to read books on photography, and so it goes.

4. A contrast with mainstream U.S. society may be instructive here. Harkness et al. (1992) point out that mainstream parents rely heavily on literacy to help

them function as parents. They regularly consult a wide array of books on child development (child-rearing manuals have been published in English for more than 500 years; Rickert, 1966) child rearing, children's health, and medical issues. "Most have a small library on the subject" (p. 175). Indeed, I would not be surprised if this volume found its way into many such libraries by mistake. The point is that in our own society, many critical adult skills are not practiced in public and hence must be acquired through more deliberate, formal means.

5. Liberia uses U.S. currency, including both bills and coins.

6. This phenomenon is widespread, especially in Africa. See Nadel (1961) on the Nupe.

7. Contrast this totally voluntary arrangement in which only fully willing and compatible teachers and pupils get together with mandatory schooling in our own society.

CHAPTER 9

1. The Kpelle, however, do not make this distinction themselves.

2. This is commonly reported. For example, "parents who wanted their children to acquire some occupational training, normally sent their children to work with craftsmen, such as potters, blacksmiths . . . who would teach them formally" (Ocitti, 1973, p. 89). Likewise, in the traditional English apprenticeship, fathers did not want to take on their own offspring as apprentices, fearing that the bonds of affection would interfere with the stern discipline that was a necessary attribute of the apprenticeship (Hanawalt, 1993; see also Goody, 1982).

3. It is curious that the several anthropologists (see Coy, 1989) who have become apprentices in the course of studying traditional crafts have not commented on the brevity of their own tutelage as compared with the norm. That is, the foreign anthropologists seem to master weaving, blacksmithing or pottery in a matter of months whereas the traditional apprenticeship lasts several years. I account for this by several factors. First, as wealthy foreign adults, the anthropologist/apprentice has high status and therefore does not have to do all the scutwork expected of an apprentice. Second, the anthropologist/apprentice starts out with well-developed learning strategies for this kind of situation. In our society, formal education analogous to apprenticeship begins at birth according to such scholars as Lave and Rogoff. Third, the anthropologist/apprentice is probably *not* attempting to master the "lore" of the chosen craft, and it is this esoteric material that must take considerable time to acquire.

4. Among the Nigerian Akwete, strict control ensures that only Akwete *women* learn to weave. If men attempt to learn to weave, "a curse called *isi otiti*

(curse of the beaten stick) would cause them impotency or death" (Aronson, 1989, p. 151).

5. The apprenticeship cases I draw on are taken from the recent ethnographic record. I could as well have included many cases from the historical record. Apprenticeship was well established in medieval England, for example. It lasted from 7 to 12 years and, by the 13th century, "The establishment of an apprenticeship contract was a matter of regulation, custom and social bonds" (Hanawalt, 1993, p. 131). Interestingly, entering an apprenticeship was ringed around with ceremony and has been likened to an "initiation ritual" (Hanawalt, 1993, p. 139).

6. The reader is referred to Buddy Bellman's (1975, 1983) thorough study of Kpelle medicine, including the process of becoming a *Zò*, something he experienced firsthand.

7. Patricia Greenfield and Jean Lave (1982) draw an interesting contrast between different weaving traditions in two distant Zinacanteco communities. In one, girls learn to weave on their own with, inevitably, a great deal of trial and error. The process looks much more like the skill learning described in the previous chapter than apprenticeship. In this village, novel designs appear with regularity. In the contrasting village, girls learn to weave under close supervision; they observe, copy, and their mistakes are instantly corrected. These girls were utterly incapable of generating patterns other than the three traditionally used in their village.

As a footnote to this footnote, I was interested to note that the conservative village was not far from San Cristobal in the Chiapas Highlands of Mexico, whereas the other village lies in Guatemala. When I visited the craft market in San Cristobal in 1993, I was puzzled to find that most of the woven work on display was produced in Guatemala and not in the immediate region. I now realize that this work—pot holders shaped like ducks, in garish colors—was quite nontraditional and more appealing to tourists. The Guatemalan enculturating routines have produced a generation of adaptive, flexible weavers.

8. An interesting example—closely parallel to those described in this chapter—is from a case study of a concert organist (the maestro) and his students (Persson, in press).

9. According to my colleague John Neeley, who has studied ceramics in Japan over extended periods, the majority of Japan's top art potters are now university trained.

10. The recent literature on apprenticeship (e.g., Greenfield & Lave, 1982) does not always tally with the points raised in this chapter. For example, in several societies all women are expected to become weavers. In these same societies, female teachers seem much more supportive and considerate of their students than

seems to be the case when the master and apprentice are male. However, I am not sure that these cases fit my conception of what an apprenticeship is.

11. A broad-based review of the initiation rite as a means of socializing children can be found in Lancy (1975b).

12. Although Bellman (1983) also collected a woman's song, whose theme was that men were callous in the treatment of children.

13. Like many aspects of bush school, there is wide disagreement on the age of initiation. Dennis (1972) says it is 18 for the Gbandes, close neighbors of the Kpelle. I do not believe that 18-year-olds would so easily acquiesce to having sometimes elderly men—the *Zò-na*—brutalize them. On the other hand, it is imperative, for bush school to have the desired effect, that "graduates" exhibit a heightened maturity. They should clearly be on the threshold of manhood. A young girl should emerge as a near-woman ready for marriage and childbearing. Hence, children much younger than 13 to 14, would not be likely candidates. The picture in Liberia has been clouded by the spread of Western influence, including public schools. Liberian politicians descended from freed slaves and, hence without tribal affiliation, have found it expedient to "join" *Poro*—often at an advanced age. Also, more and more men are paying to have their young sons (under 9) given a quickie initiation so that bush school does not interfere with their Western education. Thus, my best guess is that, traditionally, children began bush school some time between the ages of 11 and 15 and finished 3 (for girls) to 4 (for boys) years later.

14. Studstill (1979) makes the point, in his analysis of Luba initiation rites, that they reinforce the inherent class hierarchy. That is, parents and their offspring are made to kowtow to the bush school leaders, who just happen to be drawn from high-ranking members of the society. I have no doubt that this is true also for the Kpelle. *Poro* and *Sande* leaders are unquestionably the town elite.

15. For the Kpelle, that is; the *Sande* among the Mende—neighbors of the Kpelle—is well documented (Marianne Ferme, personal communication, July 1995).

16. One well-known example in the literature is the Puluwat school for navigators. Thomas Gladwin (1970), as part of an ethnography of navigation and sailing in the Caroline Islands, documented the lengthy and complex apprenticeship entered into by aspirant navigators on Puluwat Island. Puluwat Islanders are famous throughout the region for undertaking frequent long-distance canoe journeys over the open ocean, made possible by the region's several brilliant navigators. Gladwin's description of the navigators' apprenticeship more closely approximates the "formal" end of the continuum than anything I have seen in the literature on enculturation.

> Formal instruction begins on land. It demands that great masses of factual information be committed to memory. This information is detailed, specific, and potentially of

life-or-death importance. It is taught by a senior navigator to one or several students, some young, some older. Often they sit together in the canoe house, perhaps making little diagrams with pebbles on the mats which cover the sandy floor. The pebbles usually represent stars, but they are also used to illustrate islands and how the islands "move" as they pass the canoe on one side or the other. (pp. 128–129)

The star courses . . . with respect to the rising and setting of stars, which are sailed in order to get from one island to another . . . [are] taught and memorized through endless reiteration and testing. The learning job is not complete until the student at his instructor's request can start with any island in the known ocean and rattle off the stars both going and returning between that island and all the others which might conceivably be reached directly from there. (pp. 130–131)

In the past instruction was very secret. There was much magic and esoteric knowledge which could be known only by the privileged few. Some of it could be used against the navigator in sorcery if others knew it. In addition the navigational skills were and still are valuable property, . . . taught . . . only for a stiff price. (p. 129)

Despite the several ways in which young men can be deterred from entering training, of those who do undertake it . . . substantially less than half, complete the course and receive recognition. . . . (p. 128)

CHAPTER 10

1. This is written from the perspective of the 1970s. The Liberian "revolution" in 1980 and the later civil war would have brought much of this change to at least a temporary halt because change in rural Liberia is fueled primarily by cash and travel. Cash would be in much shorter supply as the war strangled the economy and travel outside one's homeland has become downright suicidal. I have found it nearly impossible to learn about the fate of my friends in Gbarngasuakwelle. All foreign civilians have been evacuated and reporters are confined to the immediate vicinity of Monrovia. Anarchy reigns.

2. This is exactly what happened to my rooster.

3. I experienced my greatest culture shock in Liberia, not in encounters with Kpelle culture but with the almost random incorporation of elements of American culture into Liberian national culture.

4. Actually, alongside the official-looking game, a uniquely local version of soccer was far more popular. There were no teams and no positions, and older boys were always careful to let younger ones have an opportunity to handle the ball. Heider (1977) describes a similar phenomenon as New Guinean Highlands children transform a game introduced through the Indonesian school system by simplifying the rules and eliminating scorekeeping and winners and losers.

5. There are frightening ironies in these notes. At the time of this study, the

native peoples of Liberia existed under the oppressive hegemony of Americo-Liberians—resettled freed slaves from the American and Caribbean colonies—for nearly 100 years. The United States had pressured the Liberian government, since the 1960s, to extend democracy and economic development opportunities to the native people—hence rural schools—with textbooks from the United States. Expectations for economic advancement were raised but never filled. There were not nearly enough jobs for all those newly schooled individuals and the Americo-Liberians didn't really want to share the pie. Hence, in 1980, a coup led by native soldiers overthrew the Americo-Liberian government and assassinated the leadership, including then President Tolbert—the last of the line stretching back to Barclay.

6. This attitude is, by no means, universal. In the several Papua New Guinean societies I studied, parents wanted their educated children to leave the village to find white-collar employment in towns so they could remit money from their regular paychecks (Pomponio & Lancy, 1986).

7. With my colleague Susan Talley, I have just finished a successful trial of "Stories and More," a CD-ROM-based automated story program in a Head Start center. Essentially, at-risk children who have not been exposed to storybooks will get an intensive dose during preschool, courtesy of a tireless, errorless, well-trained machine.

8. When researchers examine the extraordinary school success of children from some East Asian migrant communities in the United States, what they find is that the parents have wholly adopted middle-class cultural routines, including bedtime stories, dancing and music lessons, supervised study and reading times and so on (Schneider & Lee, 1990).

9. It has been empirically demonstrated that school leavers acquire an "attitude." Graves and Graves (1978) found that schooled individuals on the Cook Islands (Polynesia) were more rivalrous and less generous than those who had not been to school.

References

Adams, M. J. (1990). *Beginning to read: Thinking and learning about print.* Cambridge, MA: MIT Press.

Alford, K. F. (1983). Privileged play: Joking relationships between parents and children. In F. E. Manning (Ed.), *The world of play* (pp. 170–187). West Point, NY: Leisure Press.

Altwerger, B., Diehl-Faxson, J., & Dockstader-Anderson, K. (1985). Read-aloud events as meaning construction. *Language Arts, 62*(5), 476–484.

Anderson, A. R., & Moore, O. K. (1960). Autotelic folk models. *Sociological Quarterly 1*(4), 203–216.

Aronson, L. (1989). To weave or not to weave: Apprenticeship rules among the Akwete Igbo of Nigeria and the Baulé of the Ivory Coast. In M. W. Coy (Ed.), *Apprenticeship: From theory to method and back again* (pp. 149–162). Albany, NY: SUNY Press.

Atran, S., & Sperber, D. (1991). Learning without teaching: Its place in culture. In L. T. Landsmann, (Ed.), *Culture, schooling and psychological development* (pp. 39–55). Norwood, NJ: Ablex.

Avedon, E. M. & Sutton-Smith, B. (Eds.). (1971). *The study of games.* New York: Wiley.

Bateson, G., & Mead, M. (1942). *Balinese character.* New York: New York Academy of Sciences.

Bellman, B. L. (1975). *Village of curers and assassins.* The Hague: Mouton.

Bellman, B. L. (1983) *The language of secrecy: Symbols and metaphors in Poro ritual.* New Brunswick, NJ: Rutgers University Press.

Bergin, C., Lancy, D. F., & Draper, K. D. (1994). Parents' interaction with beginning readers. In D. F. Lancy (Ed.), *Children's emergent literacy: From research to practice* (pp. 53–78). Westport, CT: Praeger.

Biema, D. (1994, February 14). Calcutta, Illinois. *Time*, pp. 30–31.

Blacking, J. (1988). Dance and music in children's cognitive development. In G. Jahoda & I. M. Lewis (Eds.), *Acquiring culture* (pp. 91–112). London: Croom Helm.

Bledsoe, C. H. (1980). *Women and marriage in Kpelle society.* Stanford, CA: Stanford University Press.

Bloch, M. N., & Adlers, S. M. (1994). African children's play and the emergence of the sexual division of labor. In J. L. Roopnarine, J. E. Johnson, & F. H.

Hooper, (Eds.), *Children's play in diverse cultures* (pp. 148–178) Albany, NY: SUNY Press.

Blount, B. G. (1972). Parental speech and language acquisition: Some Luo and Samoan examples. *Anthropological Linguistics, 14*, 119–130.

Blurton-Jones, N. (1993). The lives of hunter–gatherer children: Effects of parental behavior and parental reproduction strategy. In M. Pererira & L. Fairbanks (Eds.), *Juveniles: Comparative socioecology* (pp. 405–426). Oxford, England: Oxford University Press.

Boyden, J. (1991). *Children of the cities.* London: Zed.

Bruner, J. S. (1975). Play is serious business. *Psychology Today, 8,* 81–83.

Cain, M. (1977). The economic activities of children in a village in Bangladesh. *Population and Development Review, 3,* 201–227.

Cazden, C. B. (1992). *Whole language plus.* New York: Teachers College Press.

Cheska, A. T. (1987). *Traditional games and dances in West African nations.* Schorndorf, Germany: K. Hofman.

Chisholm, J. S. (1980). Development and adaptation in infancy. *New Directions for Child Development, 8,* 15–30.

Chodorow, N. (1978). *The reproduction of mothering.* Berkeley: University of California Press.

Cochran-Smith, M. (1986). Reading to children: A model for understanding texts. In B. B. Schieffelin & P. Gilmore (Eds.), *The acquisition of literacy: Ethnographic perspectives* (pp. 35–54). Norwood, NJ: Ablex.

Codere, H. (1956). The amiable side of Kwakiutl life: The potlatch and the play potlatch. *American Anthropologist, 58,* 334–351.

Cole, M., Gay, J. A., Glick, J., Sharp, D. W., Ciborowski, T., Frankel, F., Kellemu, J., & Lancy, D. F. (1971). *The cultural context of learning and thinking.* New York: Basic Books.

Coy, M. W. (1989). Being what we pretend to be: The usefulness of apprenticeship as a field method. In M. W. Coy (Ed.), *Apprenticeship: From theory to method and back again* (pp. 115–135). Albany, NY: SUNY Press.

Cronk, L. (1993). Parental favoritism toward daughters. *American Scientist, 81*(3), 272–280.

Damon, W. (1995). *Greater expectations.* New York: Free Press

D'Andrade, R. G. (1984). Cultural meaning systems. In R. A. Shweder & R. A. LeVine (Eds.), *Culture theory: Essays on mind, self and society* (pp. 88–119). Cambridge, MA: Harvard University Press.

D'Andrade, R. G. (1992). Schemas and motivation. In R. G. D'Andrade, (Ed.), *Human motives as cultural models* (pp. 23–44). Cambridge, England: Cambridge University Press.

Dasen, P. R. (Ed.), (1977). *Piagetian psychology: Cross-cultural contributions.* New York: Gardner Press.

Dasen, P. R., Inhelder, B., Lavallée, M., & Retschitzki, J. (1978). *Naissance de l'intelligence chez infant baoulè de Côte d'Ivoire.* Bern, Switzerland: Hans Huber.

Das Gupta, M. (1987). Selective discrimination against female children in rural Punjab, India. *Population and Development Review, 13*, 77–100.

d'Azevedo, W. L. (Ed.). (1973). *The traditional artist in African societies.* Bloomington: Indiana Press.

Defenbaugh, L. (1989). Hausa weaving—surviving amid the paradoxes In M. W. Coy (Ed.), *Apprenticeship: From theory to method and back again* (pp. 163–179). Albany, NY: SUNY Press.

De Loache, J. S. (1984). What's this? Maternal questions in joint picture book reading with toddlers. *Quarterly Newsletter of the Laboratory for Comparative Human Cognition, 6*(4), 87–95.

De Loache, J. S., & Mendoza, O. A. P. (1985). *Joint picture book interactions of mothers and one-year old children* (Tech. Report No. 353). Urbana: University of Illinois, Center for the Study of Reading. (ERIC Document Reproduction Service No. ED 274 960)

deMarrais, K. B., Nelson, P. A., & Baker, J. H. (1992). Meaning in mud: Yup'ik Eskimo girls at play. *Anthropology and Education Quarterly, 23*(2), 120–145.

Demuth, K. (1986). Prompting routines in the language socialization of Basotho children. In B. B. Schiefflin & E. Ochs (Eds.), *Language socialization across cultures* (pp. 51–79). New York: Cambridge University Press.

Dennis, B. G. (1972). *The Gbandes: A people of the Liberian hinterland.* Chicago: Nelson Hall.

Dennis, W. (1940). *The Hopi child.* New York: Appleton Century.

Dilley, M. R. (1989). Secrets and skills: Apprenticeship among Tukolor weavers. In M. W. Coy (Ed.), *Apprenticeship: From theory to method and back again* (pp. 181–198). Albany, NY: SUNY Press.

Draper, P. (1976). Social and economic constraints on child life among the !Kung. In R. B. Lee & I. DeVore (Eds.), *Kalahari hunters-gatherers* (pp. 199–217). Cambridge, MA: Harvard University Press.

Draper, P., & Cashdan, E. (1988). Technological change and child behavior among the !Kung. *Ethnology, 27*, 339–365.

Dupont, F. (1992). *Daily life in ancient Rome.* Oxford, England: Basil Blackwell.

Edgerton, R. G. (1992). *Sick societies.* New York: Free Press.

Edwards, C. P., & Whiting, B. B. (1980.) Differential socialization of girls and boys in light of cross-cultural research. *New Directions for Child Development, 8*, 45–57.

Erchak, G. M. (1976/1977). Who is the *Zo?* A study of Kpelle identical twins. *Liberian Studies Journal, 7*(1), 23–25.

Erchak, G. M. (1977). Full respect: Kpelle children in adaptation. New Haven, CT: Hraflex Books.

Erchak, G. M. (1980). The acquisition of cultural rules by Kpelle children. *Ethos, 8*, 40–48.

Erchak, G. M. (1992). *The anthropology of self and behavior.* New Brunswick, NJ: Rutgers University Press.

Erny, P. (1981). *The child and his environment in Black Africa: An essay on traditional education* (G. J. Wanjohi, Trans.). Nairobi: Oxford University Press.

Fetterman, D . M. (1989). *Ethnography: Step by step.* Newbury Park, CA: Sage.

Field, T. M., Sostek, A. M., Vietze, P., & Leiderman, P. H. (1981). *Culture and early interactions.* Hillsdale, NJ: Erlbaum.

Firth, R. (1970). Education in Tikopia. In J. Middleton (Ed.), *From child to adult* (pp. 75–90). Garden City, NY: Natural History Press.

Fisher, E. P. (1992). The impact of play on development: A meta-analysis. *Play and Culture, 5,* 159–181.

Fortes, M. (1970). Social and psychological aspects of education in Taleland. In J. Middleton (Ed.), *From child to adult* (pp. 14–74). Garden City, NY: Natural History Press.

Friedl, E. (1992, August). Moonrose watched through a sunny day. *Natural History,* pp. 34–44.

Fulton, R. M. (1968). The Kpelle traditional political system. *Liberian Studies Journal, 1*(1) 1–19.

Fulton, R. M. (1972). The political structure and functions of Poro in Kpelle society. *American Anthropologist, 74,* 1218–1233.

Furth, H. (1966). *Thinking without language.* New York: Free Press.

Gannett News Service. (1992, August 25). Teach preschoolers more, studies say. *Salt Lake Tribune,* p. A14.

Gaskins, S. & Göncü, A. (1992). Cultural variation in play: A challenge to Piaget and Vygotsky. *Quarterly Newsletter of the Laboratory of Comparative Human Cognition, 14*(2), 31–41.

Gay, J., & Cole, M. (1967). *The new mathematics and an old culture.* New York: Holt, Rinehart & Winston.

Gerdes, P. (1988). A widespread decorative motif and the pythagorean theorem. *For the Learning of Mathematics, 8*(1), 35–39.

Gibbs, J. L. Jr. (1963). Marital instability among the Kpelle: Toward a theory of epainogamy. *American Anthropologist, 65,* 552–573.

Gibbs, J. L. Jr. (Ed.). (1988). *Peoples of Africa.* Prospect Heights, IL: Waveland Press. (Original work published 1965)

Gladwin, T. (1970). *East is a big bird.* Cambridge, MA: Harvard University Press

Golden, M. (1990). *Children and childhood in classical Athens.* Baltimore, MD: Johns Hopkins University Press.

Goldschmidt, W. (1976). *Culture and behavior of the Sebei.* Berkeley: University of California Press.

Goodenough, W. H. (1971). *Culture, language and society.* Reading, MA: Addison-Wesley.

Goodnow, J. J. (1988). Children's household work: Its nature and functions. *Psychological Bulletin, 103*(1), 5–26.

Goodnow, J. J. (1990). The socialization of cognition. In J. W. Stigler, R. A.

Shweder, & G. Herdt (Eds.), *Cultural psychology* (pp. 259–286). New York: Cambridge University Press.

Goody, E. N. (1982). *Parenthood and social reproduction: Fostering and occupational roles in West Africa.* Cambridge, England: Cambridge University Press.

Goody, E. N. (1992, December). *From play to work: Adults and peers as scaffolders of adult role skills in Northern Ghana.* Paper presented at the 91st annual meeting of the American Anthropological Association, San Francisco.

Grant, J. P. (1991). *The state of the world's children.* Oxford, England: Oxford University Press.

Graves, N. B. & Graves, T. D. (1978). The impact of modernization on the personality of a Polynesian people. *Human Organization, 37,* 115–135.

Greenfield, P. M. & Lave, J. (1982). Cognitive aspects of informal education. In D. A. Wagner & H. W. Stevenson (Eds.), *Cultural perspectives on child development* (pp. 181–207). San Francisco: W. H. Freeman

Gregor, T. (1990). Male dominance and sexual coercion. In J. W. Stigler, R. A. Shweder, & G. Herdt (Eds.) *Cultural psychology* (pp. 477–495). New York: Cambridge University Press.

Hanawalt, B. A. (1993). *Growing up in medieval London.* Oxford, England: Oxford University Press.

Harkness, S., & Super, C. M. (1986). The cultural structuring of children's play in a rural African community. In K. Blanchard (Ed.), *The many faces of play* (pp. 96–103). Champaign, IL: Human Kinetics.

Harkness, S., & Super, C. M. (1995). Culture and parenting. In M. H. Bornstein (Ed.), *Handbook of parenting.* Hillsdale, NJ: Erlbaum

Harkness, S., Super, C. M., & Keefer, C. H. (1992). Learning to be an American parent: How cultural models gain directive force. In R. D'Andrade & C. Strauss (Eds.), *Human motives and cultural models* (pp. 163–178). New York: Cambridge University Press

Harris, M. (1989). *Our kind.* New York: Harper & Row.

Heath, S. B. (1982). What no bedtime story means: Narrative skills at home and school. *Language in Society, 11,* 49–76.

Heath, S. B. (1983). *Ways with words.* Cambridge, England: Cambridge University Press.

Heath, S. B. (1986). Critical factors in literacy development. In S. deCastell, A. Luke, & K. Egan (Eds.), *Literacy, society and schooling* (pp. 209–229) Cambridge, England: Cambridge University Press.

Heath, S. B. (1990). The children of Tracton's children. In J. W. Stigler, R. A. Shweder, & G. Herdt (Eds.), *Cultural psychology* (pp. 496–519). New York: Cambridge University Press.

Heath, S. B., & Branscomb, A. (1986). The book as a narrative prop in language acquisition. In B. B. Schiefflin & P. Gilmore (Eds.), *The acquisition of literacy: Ethnographic perspectives.* (pp. 6–34). Norwood, NJ: Ablex.

Heath, S. B., & Thomas, C. (1984). The achievement of pre-school literacy for mother and child. In H. Goelman, A. A. Oberg, & F. Smith (Eds.), *Awakening to literacy* (pp. 51–72). Portsmouth, NH: Heinemann.

Heider, K. G. (1977). From Javanese to Dani: The translation of a game. In P. Stevens, Jr. (Ed.), *Studies in the anthropology of play* (pp. 72–81). West Point, NY: Leisure Press.

Henries, A. D. B. (1966). *Liberian folklore.* London: Macmillan.

Henze, R. C. (1992). *Informal teaching and learning.* Hillsdale, NJ: Erlbaum.

Herdt, G. (1990). Sambia nosebleeding rites and male proximity to women. In J. W. Stigler, R. A. Shweder, & G. Herdt (Eds.), *Cultural psychology* (pp. 366–400). New York: Cambridge University Press.

Herskovits, M. J. (1948). *Man and his works.* New York: Knopf.

Hirsch, E. D. (1987). *Cultural literacy.* Boston: Houghton Mifflin.

Hobart, A. (1988). The shadow play and operetta as mediums of education in Bali. In G. Jahoda, & I. M. Lewis (Eds.), *Acquiring culture* (pp. 113–144). London: Croom Helm.

Hogbin, I. I. (1970a). A New Guinea childhood. In J. Middleton (Ed.), *From child to adult* (pp. 134–162). Garden City, NY: Natural History Press.

Hogbin, I. I. (1970b). *The island of menstruating men.* Scranton, PA: Chandler.

Howard, A. (1970). *Learning to be Rotuman.* New York: Teachers College Press.

Inhelder, B., & Piaget, J. (1958). *The early growth of logic in the child.* New York: Norton.

Irvine, J. T. (1978). Wolof "magical thinking": Culture and conservation revisited. *Journal of Cross-Cultural Psychology, 9,* 300–310.

Jahoda, G. (1982). *Psychology and anthropology: A psychological perspective.* London: Academic Press.

Jahoda, G. (1983). European "lag" in the development of an economic concept: A study in Zimbabwe. *British Journal of Developmental Psychology, 1,* 113–120.

Johnson, N. B. (1989). Prehistoric European decorated caves: Structured earth environments, initiation, and rites of passage. In J. Valsiner (Ed.), *Child development within culturally structured environments* (Vol. 2, pp. 227–267). Norwood, NJ: Ablex.

Johnston, F. E., & Low, S. M. (1995). *Children of the urban poor.* Boulder, CO: Westview.

Katz, R. (1981). Education is transformation: Becoming a healer among the !Kung and the Fijians. *Harvard Education Review, 51*(1) 57–78.

Kelly, M. (1977). Papua New Guinea and Piaget: An eight-year study. In P. R. Dasen (Ed.), *Piagetian psychology: Cross-cultural contributions.* New York: Gardner.

Kintsch, W., & Greene, E. (1978). The role of culture-specific schemata in the comprehension and recall of stories. *Discourse Processes, 1,* 1–13.

Konner, M. (1977). Evolution of human behavior development. In P. H. Leiderman, S. R. Tulkin, & A. Rosenfeld, (Eds.), *Culture and infancy: Variations in the human experience* (pp. 69–109). New York: Academic Press.

Konner, M. (1990). The nursing knot. In *Why the reckless survive* (pp. 47–56). New York: Viking.

Kramer, S. N. (1963). *The Sumerians*. Chicago: University of Chicago Press.

Kulah, A. A. (1973). *The organization and learning of proverbs among the Kpelle of Liberia.* Unpublished doctoral dissertation, University of California at Irvine.

Lancy, D. F. (1975a). *Work, play and learning in a Kpelle town.* Unpublished doctoral dissertation, University of Pittsburgh.

Lancy, D. F. (1975b). The social organization of learning: Initiation rituals and public schools. *Human Organization, 34,* 371–380.

Lancy, D. F. (1977a). Studies of memory in culture. *Annals of the New York Academy of Sciences, 285,* 297–307.

Lancy, D. F. (1977b). The impact of the modern world on village life: Gbarngasuakwelle. *Papua New Guinea Journal of Education, 13*(1), 36–44.

Lancy, D. F. (1979). *Education research 1976–1979: Reports and essays.* Port Moresby: UNESCO/Education.

Lancy, D. F. (1979). The play behavior of Kpelle children during rapid cultural change. In D. F. Lancy & B. A. Tindall (Eds.), *The anthropological study of play: Problems and prospects* (Rev. ed., pp. 72–79). West Point, NY: Leisure Press. (Original work published 1976)

Lancy, D. F. (1980a). Becoming a blacksmith in Gbarngasuakwelle. *Anthropology and Education Quarterly, 11,* 266–274.

Lancy, D. F. (1980b). Play in species adaptation. *Annual Review of Anthropology, 9,* 471–495.

Lancy, D. F. (1980c). Speech events in a West African court. *Communication and Cognition, 13*(4), 397–412.

Lancy, D. F. (1980d). Work as play: The Kpelle case. In H. Schwartzman (Ed.), *Play and culture* (pp. 324–328). West Point, NY: Leisure Press.

Lancy, D. F. (1982). Socio-dramatic play and the acquisition of occupational roles. *Review Journal of Philosophy and Social Science, 7,* 285–295.

Lancy, D. F. (1983). *Cross-cultural studies in cognition and mathematics.* New York: Academic Press.

Lancy, D.F. (1984). Play in anthropological perspective. In P. K. Smith (Ed.), *Play in animals and humans* (pp. 295–304). London: Basil Blackwell.

Lancy, D. F. (1989). An information processing framework for the study of culture and thought. In D. Topping, V. Kobayashi, & D. Crowell (Eds.), *Thinking across cultures* (pp. 13–26) Hillsdale, NJ: Erlbaum.

Lancy, D. F. (1993). *Qualitative research in education: An introduction to the major traditions.* White Plains, NY: Longman.

Lancy, D. F. (1994a). Anthropological study of literacy and numeracy. In T. Husén & T. N. Postlewaite (Eds.), *The international encyclopedia of education* (2nd ed., pp. 3346–3453). London: Pergamon.

Lancy, D. F. (1994b). The conditions that support emergent literacy. In D. F. Lancy (Ed.), *Children's emergent literacy: From research to practice* (pp. 1–19). Westport, CT: Praeger.

Lancy, D. F. (1994c). Stimulating/simulating environments that support emergent literacy. In D. F. Lancy (Ed.), *Children's emergent literacy: From research to practice* (pp. 127–156). Westport, CT: Praeger.

Lancy, D. F. (1995, May 16). *Succor the children: A morality for the 21st century.* Utah State University Honors Lecture.

Lancy, D. F., Draper, K. D., & Boyce, G. (1989). Parental influence on children's acquisition of reading. *Contemporary Issues in Reading, 4*(1), 83–93.

Lancy, D. F., & Goldstein, G. (1982). The use of nonverbal Piagetian tasks to assess the cognitive development of autistic children. *Child Development, 53,* 1233–1241.

Langness, L. L. (1981). Child abuse and cultural values: The case of New Guinea. In J. Korbin (Ed.), *Child abuse and neglect* (pp. 13–34). Berkeley: University of California Press.

Lareau, A. (1989). *Home advantage.* New York: Falmer.

Lave, J. (1977). Tailor-made experiments and evaluating the intellectual consequences of apprenticeship training. *Anthropology and Education Quarterly, 8,* 177–180.

Lave, J., & Wenger, E. (1991). *Situated learning.* New York: Cambridge University Press.

Lebra, T. S. (1994). Mother and child in Japanese socialization: A Japan–U.S. comparison. In P. M. Greenfield & R. R. Cocking, (Eds.), *Cross-cultural roots of minority child development* (pp. 259–274). Hillsdale, NJ: Erlbaum.

Lee, R. B. (1979). *The !Kung San.* New York: Cambridge University Press.

Leighton, D., & Kluckhohn, C. (1948). *Children of the people.* Cambridge, MA: Harvard University Press.

Leis, P. (1972). *Enculturation and Socialization in an Ijaw village.* New York: Holt, Rinehart & Winston.

Lever, J. (1978). Sex differences in the complexity of children's play and games. *American Sociological Review, 43,* 471–483.

Levin, P. F. (1990). Culturally contextualized apprenticeship: Teaching and learning through helping in Hawaiian families. *Quarterly Newsletter for the Laboratory of Comparative Human Cognition 12*(2), 80–86.

LeVine, R. A. (1973). Patterns of personality in Africa. *Ethos, 1*(2), 123–152.

LeVine, R. A. (1984). Properties of culture: An ethnographic view. In R. A. Shweder & R. A. LeVine (Eds.), *Culture theory: Essays on mind, self and society* (pp. 67–87). Cambridge, MA: Harvard University Press.

LeVine, R. A. (1988). Human parental care: Universal goals, cultural strategies, individual behavior. *New Directions for Child Development, 40,* 3–11.

LeVine, R. A., & LeVine, B. (1963). Nyansongo: A Gusii community in Kenya. In B. Whiting (Ed.), *Six cultures: Studies of child rearing* (pp. 19–202). New York: Wiley.

LeVine, R. A., & White, M. I. (1986). *Human conditions.* New York: Routledge & Kegan Paul.

LeVine, S., LeVine, R. (1981). Child abuse and neglect in sub-Saharan Africa. In J. Korbin (Ed.),*Child abuse and neglect* (pp. 35–55). Berkeley: University of California Press.

Little, K. (1970). The social cycle and initiation among the Mende. In J. Middleton (Ed.), *From child to adult* (pp. 207–225). Garden City, NY: Natural History Press.

Many, J. E. (1988, April). *Interactions about text and pictures: A discourse analysis.* Paper presented at the annual meeting of the American Educational Research Association, New Orleans.

Martini, M. (1994). Peer interactions in Polynesia: A view from the Marquesas. In J. L. Roopnarine, J. E. Johnson, & F. H. Hooper (Eds.), *Children's play in diverse cultures* (pp. 73–103). Albany, NY: SUNY Press.

Mathews, H. F. (1992). The directive force of morality tales in a Mexican community. In R. D'Andrade & C. Strauss (Eds.), *Human motives and cultural models* (pp. 127–162), New York: Cambridge University Press.

McCarron, K. (1993, April 14). Professor moves the immovable to rescue the exploited. *Chronicle of Higher Education,* p. A5.

McNaughton, P. R. (1988). *The Mande blacksmiths.* Bloomington: Indiana University Press.

Mead, M. (1928). *Coming of age in Samoa* New York: Morrow.

Mead, M. (1935). *Sex and temperament.* New York: Morrow.

Miller, P. J., & Goodnow, J. J. (1995). Cultural practices: Toward an integration of culture and development. In J. J. Goodnow, P. J. Miller, & F. Kessel (Eds.), Cultural practices as contexts for development. *New Directions for Child Development, 67,* 5–16.

Milner, R. (1991, July). Alfred Russel Wallace's malaria "fit." *Natural History,* p. 53.

Murdock, G. P. (1959). *Africa: Its people and their culture history.* New York: McGraw-Hill.

Murtaugh, M. (1984). A model of grocery shopping decision processes based on verbal protocol data. *Human Organization, 45,* 243–251.

Nadel, S. F. (1961). *Black Byzantium.* London: International African Institute.

Nerlove, S. B., Roberts, J. M., et al. (1974). Natural indicators of cognitive development: An observational study of rural Guatemalan children. *Ethos, 2,* 265–295.

Nicolaisen, I. (1988). Concepts and learning among the Punan Bah of Sarawak. In G. Jahoda & I. M. Lewis (Eds.), *Acquiring culture* (pp. 193–222). London: Croom Helm.

Ninio, A., & Bruner, J. S. (1978). The achievement and antecedents of labelling. *Journal of Child Language, 5,* 5–15.

Nsamenang, A. B. (1992). *Human development in cultural context: A third world perspective.* Newbury Park, CA: Sage

Nsamenang, A.B., & Lamb, M. E. (1994). Socialization of Nso children in the Bamenda grassfield of Northwest Cameroon. In P. M. Greenfield & R. R. Cocking (Eds.), *Cross-cultural roots of minority child development* (pp. 133–146). Hillsdale, NJ: Erlbaum.

Nydegger, W., & Nydegger, C. (1963). Tarong: An ilocosbario in the Philippines. In B. Whiting (Ed.), *Six cultures: Studies in child rearing* (pp. 693–867). New York: Wiley.

Ochs, E., & Schieffelin, B. B. (1984). Language acquisition and socialization: Three developmental stories and their implications. In R. Shweder & R. L. LeVine (Eds.), *Culture theory: Essays on mind, self and society* (pp. 276–320). New York: Cambridge University Press.

Ocitti, J. P. (1973). *African indigenous education as practiced by the Acholi of Uganda.* Kampala: East African Literature Bureau.

Opie, P., & Opie, I. (1969). *Children's games in street and playground.* Oxford, England: Clarendon.

Ottenberg, S. (1989). *Boyhood rituals in an African society: An interpretation.* Seattle: University of Washington Press.

Parker, S. T. (1984). Playing for keeps: An evolutionary perspective on human games. In P. K. Smith (Ed.), *Play in animals and humans* (pp. 271–294). London: Basil Blackwell.

Persson, R. S. (in press). Studying with a musical maestro: A case study of commonsense teaching in artistic training. *Creativity Research Journal.*

Pfeiffer, J. E. (1982). *The creative explosion.* New York: Harper & Row.

Phillips, S. U. (1983). *The invisible culture.* White Plains, NY: Longman.

Piaget, J. (1951). *Play dreams and imitation in childhood.* New York: Norton.

Piaget, J. (1965). *The moral judgement of the child.* New York: Norton.

Pomponio, A., & Lancy, D. F. (1986). A pen or a bush knife: School, work and personal investment in Papua New Guinea. *Anthropology and Education Quarterly, 17*, 40–61.

Price-Williams, D., Gordon, W., & Ramirez, M. H. (1969). Skill and conservation: A study of pottery-making children. *Developmental Psychology, 1,* 769.

Purcell-Gates, V. (1994). Nonliterate homes and emergent literacy. In D. F. Lancy (Ed.), *Children's emergent literacy: From research to practice* (pp. 41–52). Westport, CT: Praeger.

Rabain-Jamin, J. (1994). Language and socialization of the child in African families living in France. In P. M. Greenfield & R. R. Cocking (Eds.), *Cross-cultural roots of minority child development* (pp 147–195). Hillsdale, NJ: Erlbaum.

Raum, O. F. (1940). *Chaga childhood.* London: Oxford University Press.

Read, M. (1960). *Children of their fathers: Growing up among the Ngoni of Malawi.* New Haven, CT: Yale University Press.

Retschitzki, J. (1989). Evidence of formal thinking in Baoulé Awélé players. In D. M. Keats, D. Munro, & L. Mann (Eds.), *Heterogeneity in cross-cultural psychology,* (pp. 234–243). Amsterdam: Swets & Zeitlinger.

Retschitzki, J. (1990). S*tratégies des jouers d'Awélé.* Paris: Harmattan.

Richards, A. I. (1956). *Chisungu*. London: Faber & Faber. (Original work published 1931)

Rickert, E. (Ed.), (1966). *The Babes' medieval manners*. New York: World.

Riesman, P. (1992). *First find yourself a good mother*. New Brunswick, NJ: Rutgers University Press.

Roberts, J. M. (1951). Three Navajo households. *Peabody Museum of Harvard University, Papers, 40*(3).

Roberts, J. M. (1964). The self-management of cultures. In W. H. Goodenough (Ed.), *Explorations in cultural anthropology* (pp. 433–454). New York: McGraw-Hill.

Roberts, J. M. (1987). Within cultural variation. *American Behavioral Scientist 31*(2), 266–279.

Roberts, J. M., Arth, M. J., & Bush, R. R. (1959). Games in culture. *American Anthropologist, 61*, 597–605.

Roberts, J. M., & Forman, M. L. (1971). Riddles: Expressive models of interrogation. *Ethnology, 10*(4) 509–533.

Roberts, J. M., & Sutton-Smith, B. (1962). Child training and game involvement. *Ethnology, 2*, 166–185.

Robinson, J. A. (1989). "What we've got here is a failure to communicate": The culture context of meaning. In J. Valsiner (Ed.), *Child development within culturally structured environments* (Vol. 2, pp. 137–198). Norwood, NJ: Ablex.

Rogoff, B. (1990). *Apprenticeship in thinking: Cognitive development in social context*. New York: Oxford University Press.

Rogoff, B., et al. (1975). Age of assignment of roles and responsibilities to children. *Human Development, 18*, 353–369.

Rogoff, B., & Lave, J. (Eds.). (1984). *Everyday cognition: Its development in social context*. Cambridge, MA: Harvard University Press.

Scheper-Hughes, N. (Ed.). (1987). *Child survival*. Dordrecht, The Netherlands: D. Reidel.

Scheper-Hughes, N. (1989). Death without weeping. *Natural History*, pp. 8–16.

Schieffelin, B. B. (1979). *How Kaluli children learn what to say, what to do and how to feel: An ethnographic study of the development of communicative competence*. Unpublished doctoral dissertation, Columbia University, New York.

Schieffelin, B. B., & Ochs, E. (Eds.). (1986). *Language socialization across cultures*. New York: Cambridge University Press.

Schieffelin, B. B. (1986). Teasing and shaming in Kaluli children's interactions. In B. B. Schieffelin & E. Ochs (Eds.), *Language socialization across cultures* (pp. 165–181). New York: Cambridge University Press.

Schildkrout, E. (1990). Children's roles, the young traders of Northern Nigeria. In J. P. Spradley & D. W. McCurdy (Eds.), *Conformity and conflict* (7th ed., pp. 221–228). Glenview, IL: Scott Foresman.

Schneider, B., & Lee, Y. (1990). A model for academic success: The school and home environment of East Asian students. *Anthropology and Education Quarterly, 12*(4), 358–377.

Schultz, W. (1973). *A new geography of Liberia.* London: Longman.

Schwartzman, H. B. (1978). *Transformations: The anthropology of children's play.* New York: Plenum Press.

Scribner, S., & Cole, M. (1973). Cognitive consequences of formal and informal education. *Science, 182,* 553–559.

Scribner, S., & Cole, M. (1981). *The psychology of literacy.* Cambridge, MA: Harvard University Press.

Serpell, R. (1993). *The significance of schooling.* Cambridge, England: Cambridge University Press.

Shweder, R. A. (1984). Preview: A colloquy of culture theorists. In R. A. Shweder & R. L. LeVine (Eds.), *Culture theory: Essays on mind, self and emotion* (pp. 1–26) New York: Cambridge University Press.

Simon, H. A. (1956). Rational choice and the structure of the environment. *Psychological Review, 63,* 129–138.

Singleton, J. (1989). Japanese folkcraft pottery apprenticeship: Cultural patterns of an educational institution. In M. W. Coy (Ed.), *Apprenticeship: From theory to method and back again* (pp. 13–30). Albany, NY: SUNY Press.

Skinner, B. F. (1963). Operant behavior. *American Psychologist, 18,* 503–515.

Smilansky, S. (1968). *The effects of sociodramatic play on disadvantaged preschool children.* New York: Wiley.

Snow, C. E., Barnes, W. S., Chandler, J., Goodman, I. F., & Hemphill, L. (1991). *Unfulfilled expectations: Home and school influences on literacy.* Cambridge, MA: Harvard University Press.

Snow, C. E., & Goldfield, B. A. (1982). Building stories: The emergence of information structures from conversation. In D. Tannen (Ed.), *Analyzing discourse: Text and talk* (pp. 127–141). Washington, DC: Georgetown University Press.

Snow, C. E., & Goldfield, B. A. (1983). Turn the page please: Situation-specific language acquisition. *Journal of Child Language, 10,* 551–569.

Spencer, F. C. (1899). *Education of the Pueblo child: A study in arrested development.* New York: Columbia University Press.

Spencer, P. (1970). The function of ritual in the socialization of the Samburu Moran. In P. Mayer (Ed.), *Socialization: The approach from social anthropology* (pp. 127–157). London: Tavistock.

Stone, R. M. (1971/1972). Menei-pelee: A musical dramatic folktale of the Kpelle. *Liberian Studies Journal, 4*(1) 31–46.

Stone, R. M. (1988). *Dried millet breaking.* Bloomington: Indiana University Press.

Strouhal, E. (1990). Life of ancient Egyptian children according to archaeological sources. In G. Beunen (Ed.), *Children and exercise* (pp. 184–196). Stuttgart, Germany: Enke.

Studstill, J. D. (1979). Education in Luba society. *Anthropology and Education Quarterly, 10*(2), 67–79.

Super, C. M., & Harkness, S. (1986). The developmental niche: A conceptualization at the interface of child and culture. *International Journal of Behavioral Development 9*, 545–569.

Sutton-Smith, B. (1977). Commentary. *Current Anthropology, 18*(2), 184–185.

Teale, W. H. (1978). Positive environments for learning to read: What studies of early readers tell us. *Language Arts, 55*, 922–932

Teale, W. H., & Sulzby, E. (1987). Literacy acquisition in early childhood: The roles of access and accommodation in storybook reading. In D. A. Wagner (Ed.), *The future of literacy in a changing world* (pp. 111–130). Oxford, England: Pergamon.

Tharp, R. G., & Gallimore, R. (1988). *Rousing minds to life.* New York: Cambridge University Press.

Thomasson, G. C. (1987). Primitive Kpelle steel making: High technology an indigenous knowledge system for Liberia's future? *Liberian Studies Journal, 12*(2), 149–164.

Tudge, J., Putnam, S., & Sidden, J. (1993). Preschoolers' activities in sociocultural context. *Quarterly Newsletter of the Laboratory of Comparative Human Cognition, 15*(2), 71–84.

Valsiner, J. (1984). Construction of the zone of proximal development in adult–child joint action. In B. Rogoff & J. Wertsch (Eds.), *Children's learning in the zone of proximal development* (pp. 65–76). San Francisco: Jossey-Bass.

Valsiner, J. (1989a). General introduction. In J. Valsiner (Ed.), *Child development in cultural context* (p 1–10). Toronto: Hogrefe & Huber.

Valsiner, J. (1989b). *Human development and culture.* Lexington, MA: Lexington Books.

Valsiner, J. (1989c). Organization of children's social development in polygamic families. In J. Valsiner (Ed.), *Child development in cultural context* (pp. 67–85). Toronto: Hogrefe & Huber.

Valsiner, J., & Hill, P. E. (1989). Socialization of American toddlers for social courtesy. In J. Valsiner, (Ed.), *Child development in cultural context* (pp. 163–179). Toronto: Hogrefe & Huber.

van Gennep, A. (1960). *Rites of passage.* London: Routledge & Kegan Paul. (Original work published 1909)

Vennum, T., Jr. (1994). *American Indian lacrosse: Little brother of war.* Washington, DC: Smithsonian Press.

Vygotsky, L. S. (1962). *Thought and language.* Cambridge, MA: MIT Press.

Vygotsky, L. S. (1967). Play and its role in the mental development of the child. *Soviet Psychology, 5*, 6–18.

Vygotsky, L. S. (1978). *Mind in society.* Cambridge, MA: Harvard University Press.

Watson-Gegeo, K. A., & Gegeo, D. W. (1986). Calling out and repeating routines among Kwara'ae children. In B. B. Schieffelin & E. Ochs (Eds.), *Language socialization across cultures* (pp. 17–50). New York: Cambridge University Press.

Watson-Gegeo, K. A., & Gegeo, D. W. (1989). The role of sibling interaction in child socialization. In P. G. Zukow (Ed.), *Sibling interaction across cultures* (pp. 54–76). New York: Springer-Verlag,.

Weisner, T., & Gallimore, R. (1977). My brother's keeper. *Current Anthropology, 18*(2), 169–180.

Welles-Nystrom, B. (1988). Parenthood and infancy in Sweden. *New Directions for Child Development, 40,* 75–96.

White, B. (1982). Child labour and population growth in rural Asia. *Development and Change, 13,* 587–610.

White, G. M. (1987). Proverbs and cultural models. In D. Holland & N. Quinn (Eds.), *Cultural models in language and thought* (pp. 151–172). New York: Cambridge University Press.

White, R. W. (1959). Motivation reconsidered: The concept of competence. *Psychological Review, 66,* 297–333.

Whiting, B. B., & Edwards, C. P. (1988). *Children of different worlds.* Cambridge, MA: Harvard University Press.

Whiting, J. W. M. (1941). *Becoming a Kwoma.* New Haven, CT: Yale University Press.

Williams, T. R. (1969). *A Borneo childhood: Enculturation in Dusun society.* New York: Holt, Rinehart & Winston.

Williams, T. R. (1983). *Socialization.* Englewood Cliffs, NJ: Prentice-Hall. (Original work published 1972)

Wilson, M. (1963). *Good company: A study of Nyakyusa Age Villages.* Boston: Beacon Press.

Wolcott, H. F. (1991). Propriospect and the acquisition of culture. *Anthropology and Education Quarterly, 22,* 251–273.

Wood, D. J., Bruner, J. S., & Ross, G. (1976). The role of tutoring in problem solving. *Journal of Child Psychology and Psychiatry, 17,* 89–100.

Zaslavsky, C. (1973). *Africa counts.* Boston: Prindle, Weber & Schmidt.

Zukow, P. G. (1989). Siblings as effective socializing agents: Evidence from central Mexico. In P. G. Zukow (Ed.), *Sibling interaction across cultures* (pp. 79–105). New York: Springer-Verlag

Author Index

Subject Index

Age-appropriate behavior, skills, 25, 27, 39, 79, 145
American culture. *See* Western society (contemporary)
Apprenticeship, 3, 10, 89, 154, 160, 163–170, 177, 178, 190, 193–196, 200, 211–213
  Master–apprentice relations, 164, 166, 167, 169, 193, 195, 211, 213

B

Blacksmithing, 3, 42, 43, 50, 61, 89, 90, 167–170, 174
Bush school, 3, 10, 13, 28, 35, 39, 40, 45, 66, 78, 124, 160, 163, 171–178, 195, 200, 213

C

Change, in children's play, 10, 109, 112, 185–189, 214
Character formation, 9, 19, 75–78, 94, 115, 118
Child bearing, 8, 12–15, 199, 201, 202, 205, 210
Child caretaking. *See* Parenting practices
Child development theory, 12, 18–23, 29, 92, 161

Child rearing. *See* Parenting practices
Children and gender, 39, 44, 74, 77, 89, 97, 98, 107, 110, 111, 127, 128, 130, 148, 149, 153, 160, 161, 172, 174, 190, 201, 208, 210
Children and economics, 12, 15, 92, 110, 145, 148, 159, 167, 201, 210
Children's acquisition of:
  Adult roles, 19, 28, 89, 90, 98, 124, 168, 169, 173, 210
  Gender appropriate, 19, 75, 76, 85, 90, 147, 172–175
  Zò, role of, 31, 70, 71, 162, 166, 170, 178, 183
  Blacksmithing, 89, 90, 161, 166–170, 178, 183, 186, 190
  Cognitive skills, including arithmetic, perception, 97, 104–106, 110, 115, 136, 158–160, 187, 194, 197
  Etiquette, social relations, 22, 23, 66, 80–83, 90, 168, 169, 205
  Farming practices, 8, 27, 52, 84, 85, 87, 103, 159–161, 190, 203
  Games, 95, 104, 105, 110–119
  Hunting and trapping, 21, 39, 84, 85, 97, 98, 146, 147, 159–161, 186
  Malaŋ game, 114–119, 186
  Marketing, 55, 156–162, 194
  Music, singing, and dancing, 28, 90, 121–124